W9-CCY-992

Promoting Sexual Responsibility

A Teen Pregnancy

Prevention Resource

for School Employees

by Eva Marx, Vicki Harrison & Kandra Strauss Riggs

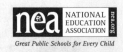

nea NATIONAL EDUCATION ASSOCIATION nea.org

Great Public Schools for Every Child

NEA PROFESSIONAL LIBRARY

NEA·HIN

NATIONAL EDUCATION ASSOCIATION
HEALTH INFORMATION NETWORK

1201 Sixteenth Street, N.W., Washington, D.C. 20036-3290

Copyright©2005 National Education Association of the United States

Printing History
 First Printing: June 2005

Note: The opinions in this publication should not be construed as representing the policy or position of the National Education Association. Materials published by HIN and the NEA Professional Library are intended to be discussion documents for educators who are concerned with specialized interests of the profession.

Library of Congress Cataloging-in-Publication Data

Marx, Eva.
 Promoting sexual responsibility : a teen pregnancy prevention resource
for school employees / by Eva Marx & Vicki Harrison & Kandra Strauss Riggs.
     p. cm.
 Includes bibliographical references.
 ISBN 0-8106-3299-3 (pbk.)
 1. Sex instruction for teenagers--United States. 2. Teenage
pregnancy—United States—Prevention. I. Harrison, Vicki, 1972- II.
Riggs, Kandra Strauss, 1976- III. Title.
 HQ57.5.A3M27 2005
 613.9'071—dc22   2005050476

1 More than 90 U.S. teens become pregnant each hour. **2** Eight out of 10 of these pregnancies are unintended. **3** Over 80 percent of these pregnancies are to unmarried teens. **4** About half of these pregnancies end in a birth, the others result in miscarriage or abortion; few teens choose adoption. **5** A sexually active teenage woman using no contraceptive over the course of a year has a 90 percent chance of becoming pregnant.

Acknowledgements

We would like to thank all of the people in schools and organizations across the country who took time out of their busy schedules to share their knowledge, experience, and resources to help make this toolkit possible.

National Education Association Health Information Network Project Staff

Jerald Newberry

Kristina Grammer

Paul Sathrum

Kandra Strauss Riggs

Reviewers/Content Advisors

Bill Albert

Sue Anderson

Bonnie Bendinksy

Karen Canova

Kate Casserly

Patricia Cheatham

Jeanette Dippo

Patti Flowers-Coulson

Debbie Gifford

Renee Grier

Bruce Hanson

Lynn Hardy

Melinda Harmon

Jennifer Henry

Chris Hoye

Nancy Hudson

Sandy Lawrence

Peggy McNabb

Linda Pickett

Barbara Sullivan

Jenny Wade

Kathy Wise

Special Thanks To:

Gregg Burrage

Rings Leighton Design Group

Co-Authors: Eva Marx

       Vicki Harrison

       Kandra Strauss Riggs

Table of Contents

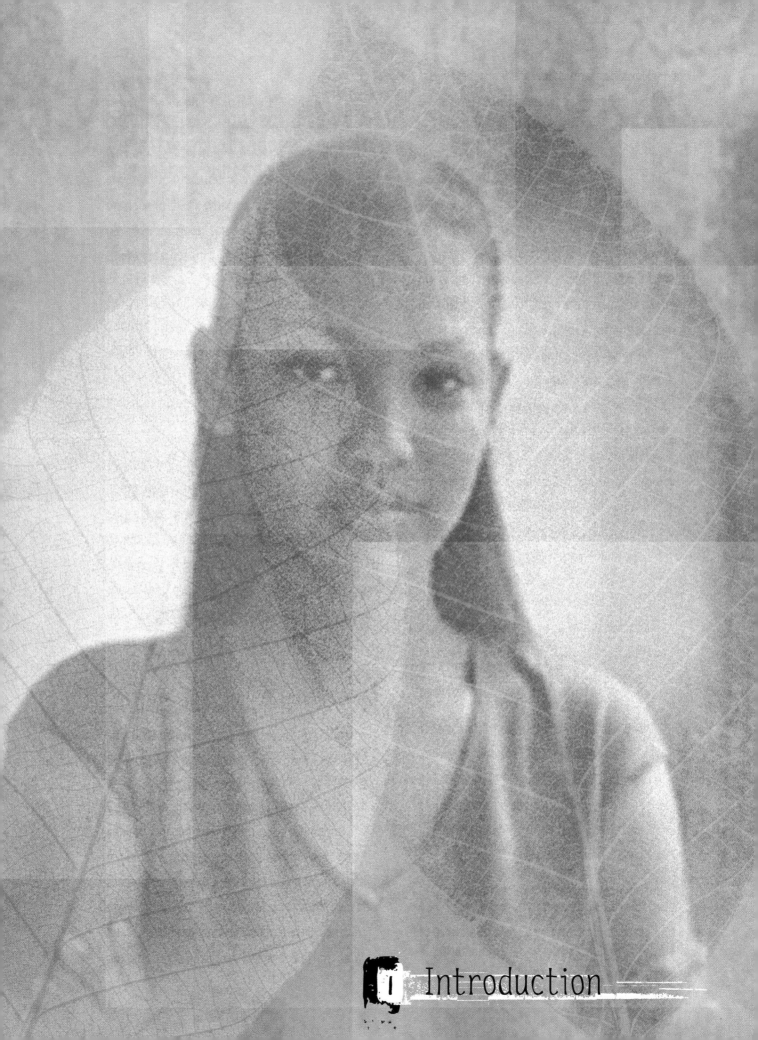

Introduction

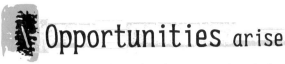Opportunities arise

every day for school personnel to help students avoid behaviors that can result in teen pregnancy as well as HIV infection and other sexually transmitted diseases (STDs). In fact, the degree to which students feel positively connected to school is strongly related to whether or not students achieve academically or engage in sexual activities that might put them at risk.

This publication offers strategies that school personnel can apply in a school setting to help young people be sexually responsible. It explores the extent and implications of teen pregnancy, ways to help young people delay sexual activity or practice safe sex, ways to help young mothers and fathers avoid second pregnancies, and resources for supporting students as they prepare for productive adulthood. It draws on current research and practice, including interviews with school-based practitioners working to prevent teen pregnancy. Some of the difficult questions it attempts to answer are:

* How pervasive is the problem of teen pregnancy?

* What can school personnel do to reduce teen pregnancy, promote responsible sexual behavior, and help students succeed?

* What are examples of effective programs and activities that schools are using?

* At what grade level should schools start to address the problem?

* What is the right program for a community?

* How do programs get organized?

Whether a school lacks a program or policy related to teen sexuality or happens to be equipped with a comprehensive program and a school-based health center, this publication is designed to provide school professionals with the most up-to-date guidance and direction on the fundamental issues surrounding teen pregnancy prevention in today's public schools.

2 The Scope of the Problem

Teen Pregnancy in the United States

Despite a decline in rates of teen pregnancy and sexual activity among youth in recent years, the United States still has the highest rate of teen pregnancy and birth in the western industrialized world—nine times as high as the Netherlands or Japan, twice as high as England and Wales or Canada. Over eight hundred thousand teenage girls get pregnant each year, most unintentionally *(The Alan Guttmacher Institute, 2000)*.

* Four out of ten young women become pregnant at least once before age 20 *(National Campaign to Prevent Teen Pregnancy, 2004)*.

* Over eight out of 10 of these pregnancies are unintended *(Henshaw, 1998)*.

* More than 80% of these pregnancies are to unmarried teens *(National Campaign to Prevent Teen Pregnancy, 2004)*.

* Over half of these pregnancies end in a birth, the others result in miscarriage or abortion; few teens choose adoption *(National Campaign to Prevent Teen Pregnancy, 2004)*.

* A sexually active teenage woman using no contraceptive over the course of a year has a 90% chance of becoming pregnant *(The Alan Guttmacher Institute, 1994)*.

HIV and Other Sexually Transmitted Diseases

STDS

Unintended pregnancy is not the only undesirable outcome of too early, unprotected sexual behaviors. Of the new cases of sexually transmitted diseases (STDs) reported each year, about three million occur in adolescents. Biologically, adolescent women may be more susceptible to STDs than older women *(The Alan Guttmacher Institute, 1994)*. The cervix of a teenage girl is more vulnerable to certain STDs than the cervix of an adult woman. And early sexual activity can actually increase the cancer risk for women. The sooner a woman starts having sex, the more likely she is to have multiple partners. That puts her at higher risk for the human papilloma virus (HPV), which has been linked to cervical cancer *(Parker-Pope, 2002)*. Other consequences of STDs for women include complications such as pelvic inflammatory disease, ectopic pregnancy, infertility, and chronic pelvic pain. Despite the fact that 15-17 year-olds account for more than 25% of new STD cases each year, 70% of sexually experienced 15-17 year-olds do not consider themselves to be at risk for STDs *(Kaiser Family Foundation/MTV/Teen People, 1999)*.

HIV/AIDS

AIDS is the sixth leading cause of death among youth ages 15-24, ranking below such injury-related causes as motor vehicle crashes, other unintentional injuries, homicide, and suicide. Evidence indicates that the presence of other STDs increases the likelihood of both transmitting and acquiring HIV infection *(U.S. Department of Health and Human Services, 2000a)*. While advances in AIDS treatment, a decrease in the number of people in this country dying from AIDS, and less media coverage of AIDS have led many to believe that the HIV epidemic is no longer of concern in the United States, the number of newly diagnosed cases of HIV infection among young people is stable at about 40,000 per year. During 1994 and 2000, 12% of HIV and AIDS cases were diagnosed in those under age 25, in the 25 states with integrated HIV/AIDS reporting. *(MMWR, 2002)*.

Women and people of color are affected disproportionately by HIV and AIDS. In 2001, 57% of HIV infections among people age 13-19 years occurred in females. African Americans and Latinos constitute approximately 15% of U.S. teenagers, yet African Americans account for 51% of AIDS cases ever reported among young people ages 13-19 and Latinos account for 20%. Of all HIV infections among 13-19 year-olds reported to date, African Americans account for 66% *(Centers for Disease Control and Prevention, 2001)*.

The Social Implications

EDUCATIONAL COSTS

Less than one-third of the young women who become mothers before the age of 18 complete high school, making teen parenthood the leading cause of high school dropout for young women. Many pregnant teens drop out of school before giving birth, putting their futures and those of their children at serious risk. Teen mothers are less likely to go on to post-secondary education or to develop the necessary skills to support themselves. Children of adolescent parents tend to be less successful academically and are 50% more likely to repeat a grade. *(The National Campaign to Prevent Teen Pregnancy, 2002)*.

HEALTH COSTS

Babies born to young mothers are more likely to be low birth-weight and to be hospitalized than are those born to older mothers. Compared to children of older parents, children of adolescent parents tend to have more health problems, receive less medical care, and experience higher rates of abuse and neglect. Adolescents who contract STDs are more likely than adult women to experience lifelong consequences such as chronic infection, ovarian abscesses, ectopic pregnancies, infertility, miscarriages, and infected babies *(American Academy of Pediatrics, 1995)*.

ECONOMIC COSTS

Teen pregnancy is costly. Nearly half a million children are born to teen mothers each year. Most of these mothers are unmarried and many end up on welfare. Male children of adolescent parents are more likely to end up in prison; females are more likely to become teen mothers. Costs include lost tax revenues and increased spending on public assistance, health care for children, foster care, and the criminal justice system. Each year the federal government alone spends about 40 billion dollars to help families that began with a teen birth *(Flinn & Hauser, 1998)*.

Factors Contributing to Teen Pregnancy

Young people are engaging in sexual activity early and, for some, often. According to the 2001 Youth Risk Behavior Survey (YRBS) *(Grunbaum et al., 2004)*:

* Over half of high school students reported that they had had sexual intercourse (61.6%) by twelfth grade.

* Over half of the young women who reported they had had sexual intercourse said that they used a condom at last intercourse. Male students were more likely than female students to report condom use (68.8% and 57.4% respectively).

* By the time they had reached twelfth grade, 22% of students reported that they had had intercourse with four or more partners.

The culture that surrounds young people, the communities in which they live, their personal knowledge, beliefs, peers, parents, school performance, and life circumstances all contribute to sexual decision making that can result in teen pregnancy. The reasons behind teen pregnancy are complex, varied, and typically interconnected. Experts have identified well over 100 antecedents to

teen sexual intercourse, poor contraceptive use, pregnancy, and childbearing *(Kirby, 2001)*. They range from individual characteristics of teens to the attitudes of their peers, their family structure, school attachment, and community setting. In addition to the antecedents discussed below, see pages 9–10 for the National Campaign to Prevent Teen Pregnancy's chart of antecedents.

Community

While race, income, and neighborhood have long been cited as key predictors of risk behaviors, demographics alone are not to blame for early sexual behavior. Some common characteristics cut across all races, incomes and classes *(Blum et al., 2000)*. The community and family with which teens live have a tremendous influence on their sexual behavior. Teens are more likely to engage in sex at an earlier age and to become pregnant in communities with less advantage and opportunity, mainly due to low expectations of them. In communities with higher levels of education, employment, and income, there may be greater opportunity and emphasis on choices that are incompatible with early childbearing, such as higher education and pursuing a career. Students at greatest risk have few positive adult role models, receive inadequate support from adults who may either not be present or may themselves be struggling for personal or economic survival, and live in neighborhoods or homes that offer little economic security or personal safety. These young people possess little hope for a successful future and little motivation to delay pregnancy or parenting *(Kirby, 1997)*.

Family

Research has shown that teens who live with both parents, feel connected to them, and are appropriately supervised are less likely to engage in unprotected sex and become pregnant *(Kirby, 2001)*. Youth who do not feel connected to family and school and do not believe that they have a promising future are less likely to have the motivation to avoid behaviors that can result in pregnancy and other undesirable health effects *(Blum & Rinehart, 1997)*. Family values and communication have an equally important impact on teen behavior. When parents express values or behaviors consistent with sexual risk-taking and early childbearing, teens are more likely to have unprotected sex and become pregnant. The same likelihood applies when a teen's older sibling enters into childbearing at an early age *(Kirby, 2001)*.

Media Messages

Teens are bombarded by media messages—advertisements, films, TV, music—that glorify sex and feature frequent sexual relationships with few or no negative consequences. The typical American child spends more than 38 hours per week—an average of nearly five-and-one-half hours a day—using media. About three hours of this time is spent watching television and one-and-a-half hours per day listening to tapes, CDs, or radio *(Kaiser Family Foundation, 1999)*. One study observed that 75% of prime time television shows included sexual content. Nearly a quarter of the couples in the programs in which sexual intercourse was depicted or strongly implied appeared to be young adults ages 18-24 and 9% appeared to be under 18. In 16% of the scenes with intercourse, the couples had just met. Not many programs encouraged responsible sexual behaviors or communicated the benefits of abstinence from behaviors frequently associated with early sexual activity such as alcohol or drug use. Few (10%) depicted safer sex and even fewer depicted abstinence. *(Kunkel et al., 1999)*. While not established as a direct precursor to teen pregnancy, most people would agree that media messages have considerable influence on teens. The media are constantly modeling sexual behaviors for the teen audience and contribute greatly to the hyper-sexualized culture today's young people are forced to navigate.

Early Initiation

"I don't think people have any idea that kids 11-or 12-years old are getting pregnant. Most of the materials are geared for older teens. These kids might not be able to read. The kids are asking me to see their friends. They are so young and naive and get involved with much older men. And we are only seeing the tip of the iceberg."
(Nurse Practitioner, Monroe County School District, FL)

A poll of children ages 8-15 and their parents showed that 68% of 8-11 year-olds said they know peers who already have boyfriends or girlfriends and 33% of 10-11 year-olds reported feeling sexual pressure *(Nickelodeon et al., 2001)*. Nationwide 7.4% of students reported initiating sexual intercourse before they were 13 years old. Black students were much more likely than white or Hispanic students to report that they had engaged in this behavior—31.8% of black male students as compared to 11.6% of Hispanic and 5.0% of white males. Among black females, 6.9% reported having had sexual intercourse before age 13, compared to 3.4% of whites *(Grunbaum et al., 2004)*.

Peer Influence

Recent data reveal that low school performance and both the quality and amount of time spent with peers are predictors of risky behaviors. Teens who spend a lot of time "hanging out" with friends, especially those engaging in risk behaviors like smoking, drinking, violence, or early sexual activity, are more likely to be involved themselves *(Blum et al., 2000)*. When teens believe their peers are having sex, whether or not this is the case, they are more likely to have sex. On the other hand, teens are more likely to use condoms or contraceptives when they believe their peers support the practice *(Bearman et al., 1999)*. Moreover, when peers are academically successful, attached to school and engage in fewer negative behaviors, a teen is less likely to become pregnant *(Kirby, 2001)*.

Clusters of Risky Behaviors

Youth who take sexual risks are more likely to engage in other risk behaviors, such as alcohol or substance abuse. Research shows that teenagers who use alcohol, tobacco, and other drugs are more likely not only to be sexually active but also to have multiple partners *(The National Center on Addiction and Substance Abuse at Columbia, 1999)*. It is believed that the relationship between substance use and sexual risk behaviors is due to a combination of factors—a general proclivity toward taking risks, an environment that supports such behaviors, and the fact that drugs and alcohol lower inhibitions and clear decision-making processes, thus increasing the incidences of risky sexual behaviors *(Kirby, 2001)*.

Psychosocial Antecedents

Of all of the external factors that contribute to the incidence of teen pregnancy, an individual's beliefs, skills, and attitudes are still the greatest predictors of sexual behavior. Teens who perceive benefits rather than costs to having sex, are unconcerned about pregnancy or STDs, and lack confidence in their ability to postpone sex are more likely to engage in sexual activity. When teens do not believe they are at risk for teen pregnancy or STDs, do not perceive that a pregnancy would have a negative effect on their lives, and are disapproving or less knowledgable about contraception, they are less likely to use contraception. Teens who initiate sex earlier, have more partners, are ambivalent about pregnancy and childbearing, and do not consistently use contraception are more likely to become pregnant *(Kirby, 2001)*.

"We have kids who feel blessed to be pregnant. It's an attempt to have someone love them. We need to change the sense of what pregnancy means." (Health Education Coordinator, Baltimore County Public Schools).

No single formula or circumstance can be used to predict a teen pregnancy, but certain factors have been shown to increase the likelihood. Some of these factors are deeply-rooted issues such as poverty and substance use—which by themselves are two of society's greatest struggles. Because it has so many complicated and overlapping antecedents, teen pregnancy is an incredibly complex problem that extends beyond the powerful but limited reach of schools. Schools alone cannot address the problem. But at the same time, young people have little hope of overcoming challenging circumstances and avoiding risky behaviors without the support of schools. As this chapter revealed, teen pregnancy has been linked to low expectations and diminished opportunities. A primary goal of schools is to increase knowledge, expectations, and opportunities for young people. The role of schools in teen pregnancy prevention is explored further in the next chapter.

Characteristics of Young Mothers

Young women who become mothers tend to:

* live in communities with high residential turnover, high poverty rates, low levels of educational attainment, and high rates of single parenthood

* have mothers or older sisters who gave birth as adolescents

* have difficulties with schoolwork

* have high rates of school absenteeism

* participate in fewer after-school and extracurricular activities

* have lower expectations for their futures

* be more likely to have been sexually abused (especially younger teen mothers)

* lack positive adult role models

* date older men

—Kirby, 1997

Important Antecedents of Adolescent Sexual Behavior, Use of Contraception, Pregnancy, and Childbearing

"+" denotes a protective factor; "-" denotes a risk factor.

COMMUNITY

Community disadvantage and disorganization

+ High level of education

- High unemployment rate

+ High income level

- High crime rate

FAMILY

Structure and economic advantage of the teenagers' families

+ Two (vs. one) parents

- Changes in parental marital status

+ High level of parents' education

+ High parental income level

Positive family dynamics and attachment

+ Parental support and family connectedness

+ Sufficient parental supervision and monitoring

Family attitudes about and modeling of sexual risktaking and early childbearing

- Mother's early age at first sex and first birth

- Single mother's dating and cohabitation behaviors

+ Conservative parental attitudes about premarital sex or teen sex

+ Positive parental attitudes about contraception

- Older sibling's early sexual behavior and age of first birth

PEER

Peer attitudes and behavior

+ High grades among friends

- Peers' substance use and delinquent and non-normative behavior

- Sexually active peers (or perception thereof)

+ Positive peer norms or support for condom or contraceptive use

Continued on next page.

Continued from page 13.

Important Antecedents of Adolescent Sexual Behavior, Use of Contraception, Pregnancy, and Childbearing

"+" denotes a protective factor; "-" denotes a risk factor.

PARTNER

Partner attitudes

+ Partner support for contraception

TEEN

Biological antecedents

- Older age and greater physical maturity
- Higher hormone levels

Ethnicity

+ Being white (vs. black or Hispanic)

Attachment to and success in school

+ Good school performance
+ Educational aspirations and plans for the future

Attachment to religious institutions

+ Frequent religious attendance

Problem or risk-taking behaviors

- Tobacco, alcohol, or drug use
- Problem behaviors or delinquency
- Other risk behaviors

Emotional distress

- Higher level of stress
- Depression
- Suicide ideation

Characteristics of relationship with partners

- Early and frequent dating
- Going steady, having a close relationship
- Greater number of romantic partners
- Having a partner 3 or more years older

Sexual abuse

- History of prior sexual coercion or abuse

Sexual beliefs, attitudes, and skills

+ Conservative attitudes toward premarital sex
+ Greater perceived susceptibility to pregnancy, STDs/HIV
+ Agreement with importance of avoiding pregnancy, childbearing, & STDs
+ Greater knowledge about contraception
+ More positive attitudes about contraception
+ Greater perceived self-efficacy in using condoms or contraception

Kirby, D. (2001). **Emerging Answers:** Research Findings on Programs to Reduce Teen Pregnancy. Washington, DC: National Campaign to Prevent Teen Pregnancy.

3 The Role of Schools

The Link Between Teen Pregnancy and Educational Achievement

"Children who suffer from violence, hunger, substance abuse, too early pregnancy, depression, and hopelessness are not healthy children. Unhealthy children are children with impaired learning."
(Lavin, Shapiro, & Weill, 1992).

Public schools serve approximately 50 million children for 13 of their most developmentally critical years—the same years when risk behaviors for teen pregnancy are established. The link between teen pregnancy and school performance is undeniable. Parenthood is a leading cause of high school dropout among teen girls *(National Association of State Boards of Education, 1998)*. Children of teen mothers are more likely to be less academically successful and are 50% more likely to repeat a grade than other children *(Maynard, 1996)*. Low academic achievers who are pessimistic about their future and feel a sense of failure in school are more likely to become pregnant. In fact, half of teen mothers drop out of school before becoming pregnant *(Manlove, 1998)*. In turn, students who are pregnant or parenting will be less likely to have the motivation, time, or energy to achieve academically or stay in school.

Academic involvement is also linked closely to teen pregnancy because of its protective properties. A relatively higher grade point average has been identified as a protective factor for delaying sexual involvement and reducing pregnancy *(Blum & Rinehard, 1997)*. Furthermore, teens are less likely to begin having sex if they feel "connected" to their school, get along with teachers and students, and feel that teachers treat students fairly *(Blum, McNeely, & Rinehart, 2002)*. A program designed to help fifth-graders achieve academically and avoid drug use also had the unanticipated effect of lowering teen pregnancy and sexually transmitted disease rates even though sexuality education was not included in the program *(Lonczak et al., 2002)*. According to one researcher *(Andersen, 2002)*, "These results fit with our theory that if children become bonded and committed to achieving in school during the elementary grades, they are less likely to risk that bond by engaging in behavior that puts their future success at risk." Clearly, improving the educational achievement of all students, particularly those at high risk of school failure, is a critical teen pregnancy prevention strategy *(Council of Chief State School Officers, 1999)*.

Partners in Progress: The Education Community and Preventing Teen Pregnancy offers ideas on ways the education community can help prevent teen pregnancy without sacrificing its core mission of education. The brochure can be downloaded from The National Campaign to Prevent Teen Pregnancy website at http://www.teenpregnancy.org.

Prevention Strategies for Schools

The National Campaign to Prevent Teen Pregnancy (1999) suggests five strategies that schools can pursue to play a role in teen pregnancy prevention:

* Promote educational success and provide an enhanced sense that life holds positive options.

* Help youth create and maintain strong connections to parents and other adults.

* Provide knowledge, reinforce positive social norms, and enhance social skills through various types of abstinence or sexuality education.

* Offer contraceptive services (either in school or nearby) or make referrals for them.

* Carry out multiple approaches through school/community partnerships.

Teen pregnancy is a complex problem with no single solution. Since every school has different staff, students, resources, and values that influence its operation, each school will want to address the issue in its own way. Below are descriptions of several different approaches. Some can be implemented inside the classroom and others by partnering with families and the larger community.

Youth Development Programs

"Youth development" describes activities that enhance life options for adolescents rather than targeting a particular behavior such as early sexual activity or substance abuse. These programs emphasize strengthening family, school, and community connections; improving adolescents' life skills and sense of competence; and increasing students' opportunities by identifying and building upon their assets. Such an approach involves life skills education, personal values assessment and development, communication and refusal skills development, promotion of education and career goals, and exposure to volunteer activities or extracurricular involvement within the community, such as service learning and after-school programs that complement school-based activities *(Washington State Department of Health, 1999).*

Youth development activities that strengthen students' sense of self-worth, connectedness, and hope for the future can be incorporated into many aspects of the school program. Creating an environment that supports healthy development; offering after-school programs, including sports; and establishing positive relationships between youth and staff are examples of teen pregnancy prevention strategies that follow the youth development model. Youth development is an ideal approach, but requires the understanding, support, and participation of the entire school community. The programs need to be tailored to the values, needs, and resources of the community in which they reside. Start-up efforts may be modest but the ultimate goal needs to be long-term and multidimensional. Specific examples of youth development programs appear throughout this chapter.

Classroom Instruction

Sexuality education curricula vary in content, duration, target age, and philosophy (from family-life and reproductive anatomy to an abstinence-only message to comprehensive programs that concentrate on life-long sexual health). Many are designed to prevent or reduce sexual risk-taking behaviors. School-based sexuality education can also occur in the form of prevention messages and health facts woven throughout instruction on other academic subjects. Chapter 5 provides examples of sexuality education strategies and programs.

Programs for Pregnant and Parenting Teens

Teens who are pregnant or parenting are at high risk for not finishing school and for having a second pregnancy. To be truly effective, school-based prevention efforts cannot overlook this population, no matter the size. Pregnant and parenting teens need specialized attention from school staff to help them stay in school and avoid second pregnancies. See chapter 9 for specific prevention strategies for working with this population.

School Climate

When people walk into a school that supports youth development they sense positive energy. These schools are places where students feel valued, safe, connected, and supported.

Administrators are concerned about the physical, social, and emotional well-being of students and staff, are attentive to health issues, and have respect for the impact of health on learning. School personnel are committed to students' academic success and believe that students are competent and able to achieve. Teachers are prepared to meet the needs of diverse learners and are responsive to students and parents. Students with special needs are equally valued and not isolated from other student activities.

In these schools, expectations are clear and students feel they are treated fairly. Parents and the community promote and model respectful behavior and communicate the value of education to students. Students develop a positive attitude toward themselves and others. Creating such an environment requires the involvement of everyone in the school—administrators; teachers; office, custodial, maintenance, and transportation staff; school nurses, counselors, psychologists, social workers, and other pupil services professionals; food services staff; parents; and students. Every member of the school community serves as a role model by being supportive and respectful of students, fellow staff members, and families *(Marx, Wooley, & Northrop, 1998)*.

After-School Programs

Students who participate in after-school programs are 37% less likely to become teen parents than students who do not *(U.S. Department of Health & Human Services, 1995)*.

Structured after-school programs reduce students' unsupervised discretionary time and consequently decrease opportunities to engage in sex and other risky activities. After-school programs give students constructive options by offering educational enrichment and creative recreational opportunities in a safe, healthy setting. Students can develop relationships with caring, competent, consistent adults who serve as mentors and role models.

Common Characteristics of After-School Programs

* encourage parent and community involvement with students

* promote community and youth service opportunities

* provide nutritious snacks or meals for students

* sponsor recreational activities and organized sports

* provide counseling services for students

* teach conflict-resolution skills
  (National Governors' Association, 2000)

Schools can support after-school programs by providing space, access, transportation, staff, management, or other resources. School day staff can advocate for the establishment and maintenance of after-school programs and encourage students to participate. School day staff can communicate, cooperate, and collaborate with after-school staff to integrate learning and enrichment activities by linking school-day and after-school curricula. They can collaborate to ensure continuity in learning by making the after-school program relevant to the school day.

Day staff and after-school teachers can meet regularly to discuss the social and academic status of participating students. Day staff can assist after-school staff by making arrangements to use facilities such as computer labs and recreational equipment. In some schools after-school staff attend school faculty meetings and share space (U.S. Department of Education & U.S. Department of Justice, 2000).

Mentors and Role Models

Lack of positive adult role models is a factor associated with early sexual behavior among teens. Young people need at least one strong, dependable adult in their lives. In an ideal world this responsibility would not fall on school personnel. Unfortunately, not all students have homes that offer such support. In too many cases, parents are not providing their children with adequate attention, skills, and information. When families do not or cannot provide sustained, caring relationships, school personnel such as teachers, school counselors, social workers, coaches, school nurses, and other staff are left to fill

The U.S. Departments of Education and Justice produced a guide for superintendents, principals, parents, communities, employers, local governments, and faith communities who want to start or expand after-school programs. *Working for Children and Families: Safe and Smart After-School Programs* outlines recent research, resources, and information on promising efforts. The guide is available on-line at http://www.ed.gov/pubs/SafeandSmart/index.html

this gap. Young people respond positively to adult role models and mentors who provide support, set limits, and have high expectations for them.

Adults can assist with homework, goal setting, development of life skills, and practicing appropriate social behaviors. They can be companions to teens and take them to sports functions, restaurants, and movies. School staff can develop positive relationships with students, either within the school setting or through a more formal arrangement with a faith-based program or a youth-serving organization such as the YMCA, YWCA, Urban League, Girl Scouts, Boys and Girls Clubs, Girls, Inc., or 4H.

Service Learning

School personnel can also link students to service learning opportunities. Service learning —or community service—helps students develop competencies, build confidence, learn about life career options, and feel connected with their communities. Students can bag supplies at local food banks, clean and refurbish streets, or walk dogs for the humane society. They can work with community agencies such as hospitals, nursing homes, senior citizen programs, or child care centers under supervision of the organizations' staff. Some teachers incorporate service learning opportunities into their curricula and provide time during class for students to report on their experiences. An evaluation of service learning programs shows that, while the youth are participating, the programs may have some of the strongest evidence of any intervention for reducing teen pregnancy rates *(Kirby, 2001)*.

Asset Development

The Search Institute in Minneapolis has developed a framework of 40 external and internal developmental assets that appear to help students perform well academically and avoid behaviors that put them at risk *(Benson, Galbraith, & Espeland, 1998)*. These assets, which the developers regard as critical for young people's growth and development, offer benchmarks for positive child and adolescent development and define roles that families, schools, congregations, neighborhoods, youth organizations, and others in communities can play in shaping young people's lives.

The 20 external developmental assets focus on young people's experiences with the people and institutions in their lives. Examples are:

* Support, care, and love from their families,

neighbors, and the organizations and institutions that can provide positive, supportive environments

* A sense of empowerment, including opportunities to contribute to others and feeling safe, secure, and valued by their community

* Clear boundaries and expectations, i.e., knowing what is expected of them

* Using time constructively

Twenty internal qualities that guide choices and create a sense of centeredness, purpose, and focus include:

* Commitment to learning

* Positive values to guide their choices

* Skills and competencies to make positive choices, build relationships, and succeed in life

* Positive identity, i.e., a strong sense of their own power, purpose, worth, and promise.

To learn more about the Search Institute's approach visit *http://www.search-institute.org/*

Physical Activity

Physical activity, including sports, may be an untapped resource for teen pregnancy prevention. Physical activity can have a positive impact on students, whether or not they are athletically gifted. Studies among adolescents consistently relate physical activity to higher self-esteem and less anxiety and stress.

Teen Outreach,

a youth development program targeting youth ages 12-17, combines volunteer community service opportunities, such as work as aides in hospitals or nursing homes, participation in walkathons, and peer tutoring, with structured discussions about life options. The program has been found to reduce substantially rates of teen pregnancy, course failure, school suspension, and school dropout (Allen, Philliber, Herrling, & Kuperminc, 1997). It can be offered
(1) in-school and integrated with core subjects,
(2) as an in-school elective,
(3) as part of an after-school program, or
(4) by a community agency. Information about the program is available from:

The Cornerstone Consulting Group, Inc., One Greenway Plaza, Suite 550, Houston, TX 77046, Phone: (713) 627-2322
Website: http://www.cornerstone.org/

Moreover, a national survey found that low levels of physical activity were associated with high-risk behaviors such as cigarette smoking and marijuana use. Schools can provide opportunities for participation in physical activity through physical education classes, recess, and links with community recreation programs in addition to intramural and interscholastic sports programs.
According to the National Association for Sport

and Physical Education, well-implemented physical education programs also contribute to students' self-discipline and provide them with opportunities to assume leadership, cooperate with others, and accept responsibility for their own behavior *(Bogden, 2000)*.

Student athletes are generally more likely than students who do not participate in athletics to have plans for college after high school graduation. Improving or maintaining their athletic skills can increase their chances for an athletic scholarship and contribute to a well-rounded student life. Pregnancy or involvement with a pregnancy can jeopardize an athlete's individual performance as well as her or his team's success. Many female high-school athletes report higher grades and standardized test scores and lower dropout rates *(The President's Council on Physical Fitness and Sports, no date)*. Athletes tend to have more positive body concepts and greater self-esteem. Participation in sports can help them become more assertive and better equipped to negotiate decisions such as whether or not to have sex or use contraceptives. Sports can provide a venue for adults to interact on a regular basis with young people in supportive ways. Coaches, teachers, and health care professionals can develop relationships with young athletes and support them in avoiding risky behaviors.

Girls who participate in sports typically feel connected and competent. Female athletes develop close-knit social networks, offering peer support and positive relationships. Sports build girls' confidence, sense of physical empowerment, and social recognition within the school and the community. While there may be no causal relationship, girls who participate in sports report later initiation of intercourse and, when they do become sexually active, they are more likely to use a condom than those not involved with sports. They report lower pregnancy rates and engage in sexual intercourse less frequently. African-American, Caucasian, and Latina female athletes alike experience a lower rate of pregnancy than those who do not participate in sports. Girls may be using self-reliance and social status gained through athletic participation to resist social pressures to exchange sex for approval or popularity *(Sabo et al., 1998)*.

Students Supporting Students

Schools should not overlook the roles that students can play in pregnancy prevention activities and ways that school staff can advise and encourage students participating in these activities. Teens can provide valuable insights on student response to program activities and can help to recruit other teens. With support from peer educators, peer support groups can meet regularly to discuss issues and concerns in a supportive, non-threatening atmosphere. Older students can become peer leaders and teach health-related classes to younger students. Students can be involved in a variety of other activities such as health fairs or teen concerts as well as peer education and presentations. Students engaged in programs such as these provide a support system for each other, while developing self-esteem and leadership skills.

A Coordinated Approach

Some districts find that teen pregnancy prevention strategies are most effectively implemented in the context of a coordinated school health program (CSHP). CSHPs include the academic support services that are so important for helping students avoid risky behaviors, including those that result in pregnancy. They address factors such as nutrition; safety; social, emotional, and behavioral disorders; and physical activity— all of which influence educational concerns such as student attendance, attentiveness, behavior, persistence, and achievement. CSHPs involve the entire school community and commonly include the following components: health education; physical education; nutrition services; health services; counseling, psychological, and social services; healthy school environment; health promotion for staff; and family/community involvement.

A well-functioning CSHP program incorporates policies that create a safe physical and positive psychosocial environment for students and staff; a team that includes key school staff; classroom activities that prepare students for healthy, productive lives; access to health care and services, nutritious meals and opportunities for physical activity; and family and community involvement *(Marx,*

Wooley, & Northrop, 1998). School personnel are engaged in the program's development and maintenance. They understand how the program contributes to the health and welfare of the school community and know to whom to turn when they encounter a situation that requires referral or other specialized professional intervention. In such programs, the health educator, the school nurse, the school counselor, and other school personnel are aware of what each is doing, resulting in more effective use of resources through reduced duplication, more targeted efforts, and increased sharing of materials and funding.

Coordinated school health programs share many goals with education reform. Both seek to improve school performance, address causes of underachievement, and develop productive, capable students. They aim to promote family and community involvement, empower teachers, strengthen professional development, provide locally determined programs and policies, and consolidate resources so that they are used more effectively and efficiently *(Education Development Center, 1999)*.

Coordinated school health programs support and enhance the protective factors upon which youth development programs focus— connections with family, school, and community. CSHPs can include caring, supportive peer or adult mentors and consistent positive health-related messages supported through communication among school personnel, families, and community members. A CSHP can contribute to a student's sense of well-being through its policies, to her or his feelings of self-worth through opportunities for community service, and to competence and mastery through health education and physical education *(Fetro, 1999)*.

The Centers for Disease Control and Prevention funds selected states to develop agency partnerships at the state level to foster the development of coordinated school health programs in schools and districts. Many national organizations, including NEA, work with their constituencies to promote coordinated school health programs. Most schools and districts have elements of the components in place. These components can function more effectively when coordi-

nated with the support of a designated coordinator and the involvement of an advisory committee. Chart I, Inventory of School and Community Programs, Activities, and Services to Prevent Teen Pregnancy (on Page 148) can help identify the activities that already exist in a school or district, which components of a coordinated school health program are involved, and gaps that might be addressed. Chart II, How We Can Support Teen Pregnancy Prevention, *(see page 149)* can help school personnel identify how they can contribute to these activities. Page 26 has resources that can help school personnel find out more about how to establish a coordinated school health program in their school or district.

Resources for learning more about coordinated school health programs and how to implement them include:

▶ *Schools and Health: Our Nation's Investment,* an Institute of Medicine report, is available from the National Academy Press, 2101 Constitution Avenue, Washington, DC 20055; (800) 624-6242. This book provides an overview of school health programming and recommendations for strengthening activities to improve the health and academic success of students.

▶ *Health Is Academic: A Guide to Coordinated School Health Programs,* edited by Eva Marx and Susan F. Wooley with Daphne Northrop, is available from Teachers College Press, P.O. Box 20, Williston, VT 05495-0020; (800) 575-6566. This book discusses the importance of health programs in support of student health and achievement and describes the roles of school personnel.

▶ *Talking About Health Is Academic: Six Workshop Modules for Promoting a Coordinated Approach to School Health* provides scripts and overhead masters for developing programs. It is available from Teachers College Press, P.O. Box 20, Williston, VT 05495-0020; (800) 575-6566.

▶ *Step by Step to Health Promoting Schools: A Guide to Implementing Coordinated School Health Programs in Local Schools and Districts* by Joyce V. Fetro, available from ETR Associates, (800) 321-4407 or http://www.etr.org, presents information and worksheets for program development.

▶ *Improving School Health: A Guide to the Role of the School Health Coordinator* and *Improving School Health: A Guide to School Health Councils,* available from local chapters of the American Cancer Society, are designed to help volunteers work with schools to establish school health programs.

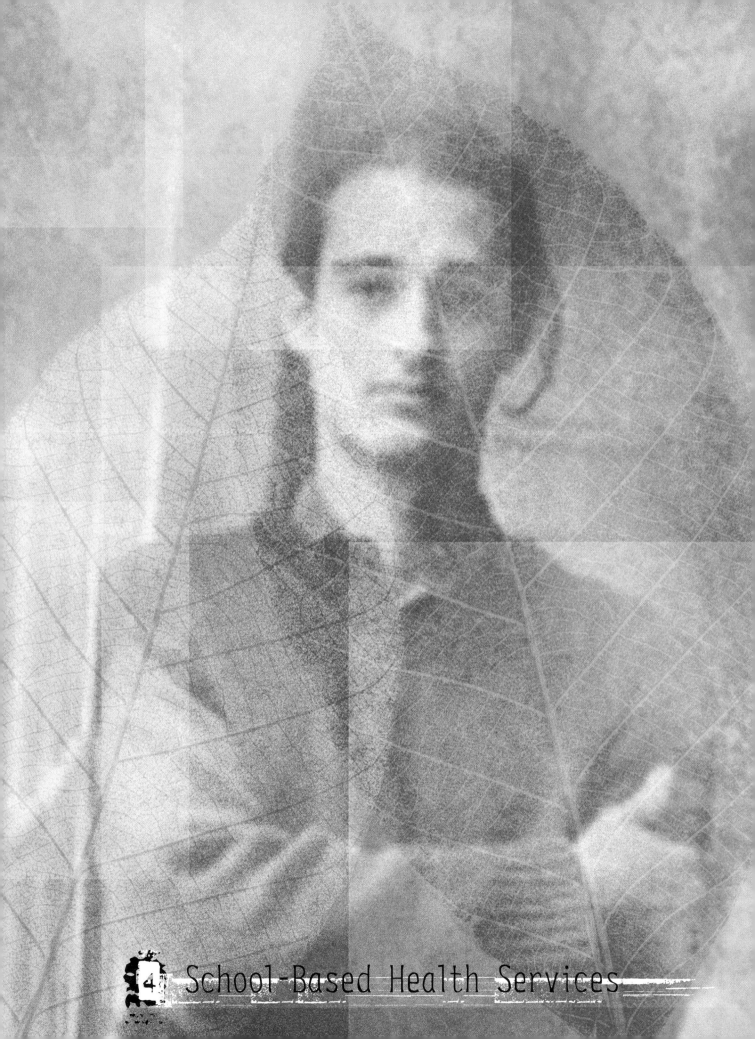

School-based health

services can provide a range of supports including counseling; pregnancy testing; breast, gynecological, and testicular exams; age-appropriate sexuality education; and screening and treatment for STDs.

The School Nurse

The school nurse is often the only health care provider at the school site on a regular basis and, as such, plays an essential role. There are approximately 58,000 registered nurses employed as school nurses in the U.S. School nursing services are mandated in 19 states *(National Association of School Nurses, 2002)*. Nurses make physical and mental health assessments, develop health care plans, interpret health care needs to school personnel, and collaborate with other school professionals such as counselors, psychologists, and social workers *(Institute of Medicine, 1997)*. The school nurse can provide information and counseling about lifestyle choices that can motivate students to avoid behaviors that put them at risk. They can provide this information to individuals, groups, classrooms, or the entire student body. Formal classroom instruction provided by the school nurse can contribute to a healthy lifestyle and increase the likelihood that students will use the services that the school nurse provides. Students may come to the nurse with a minor physical complaint and share concerns about other issues, such as a relationship. The

school nurse might be the first person to whom a student discloses a concern about a possible pregnancy. The nurse can counsel the student about risks and safety, determine whether the student is indeed pregnant, and, if so, make referrals for care. They often have referral agreements with local public health clinics or community family planning clinics. School nurses sometimes assist in the development of family life education programs and do prevention counseling with students and parents about reproductive health issues, HIV, and STDs. As described in Chapter 9, school nurses can also play a major role in programs for pregnant and parenting teens. They often provide nutrition and exercise counseling for pregnant teens, as well as conduct parenting classes and support groups.

School-Based Health Centers

Approximately 1,500 schools house school-based health centers that provide a range of services, including diagnosis, treatment and referral for illnesses, immunizations, physical examinations, and mental health counseling. Physical and mental health issues are often interconnected, especially during puberty. By offering physical and mental health services in the same location, school-based health centers are prepared to offer comprehensive care.

Students like school-based health centers because they are on campus and easily accessible, center staff are likely to be familiar with the school culture, and students are assured of confidentiality. School-based health centers give convenient, age-appropriate health care, particularly in areas where health care might be scarce or children are uninsured or underinsured. Students may reveal a problem related to sexual activity during a medical visit. About three-quarters of school-based health centers offer birth control counseling; and almost 9 out of 10 provide pregnancy testing. Many have referral agreements with community family planning clinics or health department programs that can assist youth who need services (Dailard, 2000).

In some districts school-based health centers serve school staff as well. Teachers and administrators who are enrolled become excellent sources of referral. School personnel in schools with school-based health centers, need to find out what services are provided and how center staff can assist them. Many centers hold open houses to familiarize school staff, families, and students with what they offer (Hurwitz & Hurwitz, 2000).

Principals can encourage teachers, counselors, and other school personnel to make appropriate referrals. They could organize an orientation for school staff to meet health center staff to promote understanding and reduce conflict for occasions

such as when a student needs to leave class to keep a health center appointment. Health education teachers, school social workers, counselors, and physical education instructors, in particular, can exchange information and plan joint activities with school-based health center staff, including faculty training and classroom presentations.

School boards must approve the decision to host a health center. Districts often provide school-based health centers with in-kind support such as space, renovation,

Action Steps:

1. If your school or district has a school-based health center, find out what services it provides. Ask: What reproductive health services are included? How do these complement other school pregnancy prevention activities or how could they?

2. Work with the administration and other staff to educate the school community about school-based health center services.

3. Join the school-based health center community advisory board.

4. If your school or district does not have a school-based health center, work with others in the community to determine whether such services are needed and, if so, begin to work towards its establishment.

security, and janitorial services but do not usually fund centers with district revenues. The school and the center sign a contract or memorandum of understanding that ensures compliance with district policies and spells out issues of responsibility, liability, and levels of service. A community advisory board that includes medical and social service providers, school board members, parents, civic leaders, clergy, and financial supporters participates in policy and planning and gives support and feedback. As a member of the community, a school employee could join the board as an advocate for students and staff. In Evanston, Illinois the advisory board was instrumental in convincing the school board to include reproductive health among the center's services *(Hurwitz & Hurwitz, 2000)*.

Resources for Developing School-Based Services

Advocates For Youth's Guide to Programs for School-Based and School-Linked Health Care includes information on how to plan, fund, operate, and expand school-based and school-linked health centers. Website: http://www.advocatesforyouth.org/publications.

Contact the National Assembly on School-Based Health Care at http://www.nasbhc.org **or** 202-286-8727 **for information about resources and program activities.**

Visit the Center for Health and Health Care in Schools website at http://www.healthinschools.org

Condom Availability Programs

Among the 34.3% of sexually active students in the U.S. in 2003, 63% reported that either they or their partner had used a condom during last sexual intercourse *(Grunebaum et al., 2004)*. Condoms offer sexually active youth a number of benefits:

1) highly effective birth control (correct use can result in 97% effectiveness; average use, 84%) *(Alan Guttmacher Institute, 1998)*

2) decrease transmission of some STDs

3) availability without prescription

4) minimal side effects

5) a way for males to take responsibility for birth control and STD prevention

Factors that influence condom use are access, availability, confidentiality, embarrassment, partner attitude, perception of risks for pregnancy and infection, and cost (Advocates for Youth, 1997; American Academy of Pediatrics, 1995).

More than 400 schools allow condoms to be made available in the school building through school counselors, nurses, teachers, principals, other school personnel, vending machines, or baskets (Advocates for Youth, 1997). Program requirements, which are generally dependent upon community choices, range from no restrictions to requiring counseling by health care providers or parental permission before students can obtain condoms. Acceptance of condom availability programs by parents has been high. In schools where parent permission is required, less than 2% have submitted written denials of permission (American Academy of Pediatrics, 1995). Supporters of condom availability in schools recommend that this activity be offered in conjunction with comprehensive health education as part of a coordinated school health program (Advocates for Youth, 1997; American Academy of Pediatrics, 1995). More than eight out of ten parents (85%) feel that schools should teach how to use condoms as well as how to talk with partners (Kaiser Family Foundation, 2000b). Studies of schools with health clinics and condom availability programs have consistently shown that providing condoms or other contraceptives through schools does not increase sexual activity (Kirby, 2001).

Studies comparing students at schools that made condoms available with those at schools that did not found that fewer students at schools making condoms available reported ever having had sexual intercourse than students at schools where condoms were not available. Moreover, schools making condoms available were more likely to teach students how to use them properly, students at those schools were more likely to have received information about HIV/AIDS, and students at schools with condom programs were no more likely than others to say that condoms were easily available, even though they were more likely to use them (Blake, Ledsky, & Goodenow, 2003).

Referrals

From time to time students ask questions or make statements that suggest the need for follow-up with a health or mental health professional. These can emerge at any time—during an athletic event, in the course of after-school activities, as part of a classroom discussion, on the school bus, or in the cafeteria. Sometimes students will confide in a trusted teacher or other staff member about a personal issue. At other times school personnel may observe behaviors that suggest students are engaging in or considering behaviors that could put them at risk. School personnel need to be aware of and sensitive to students' behaviors and, when appropriate, help them understand the consequences of their actions.

School personnel who have close relationships with one or more students can make themselves available to listen and talk. However, they should not try to assume the role of a mental health or social service professional. When they see a student doing something that is of concern or hear something that they feel is beyond their expertise, they can say something like, "Look. I am really worried about (what you are doing or what I have heard)" and refer him or her to a counselor or other professional who can help *(Secrist, 2000)*.

Family life and health education teachers can increase the likelihood that students will seek out needed services by inviting school nurses, counselors, and psychologists to their classes to describe available services. Schools that have coordinated school health programs often have methods for teachers to consult with other professional staff when they need to seek advice or a referral source for a student.

Confidentiality

Confidentiality is of particular concern when dealing with issues related to sexual behaviors and pregnancy. For instance, is a school nurse authorized to perform a pregnancy test on a student? If positive, can the results be shared with the student's parents without the student's consent? Students' needs for

support, services, and special academic considerations require teachers, parents, school nurses, mental health professionals, physicians, school administrators, and other pupil services personnel to communicate and collaborate. Determining what information should be shared and what should be kept confidential is not always easy. Laws and policies can be unclear or inconsistent, communication may be difficult, or staff may be inadequately prepared in the practices necessary for protecting student confidentiality *(National Task Force on Confidential Student Health Information, 2000)*.

For clarity on responding to questions such as those posed above, every district needs to establish policies and standard procedures for protecting confidentiality related to student health information. Federal and state law as well as community values need to inform policy development. As required by the Health Insurance Portability and Accountability Act *(HIPAA)*, the Standards for Privacy of Individually Identifiable Health Information (the Privacy Rule) apply to the information collected by health care providers, including those who work in schools. A school that employs a school nurse or other provider is subject to the regulations of HIPAA if they engage in certain financial and administrative transactions *(U.S. Department of Health and Human Services, 2000b, 2002)*.

However when it comes to the rights of parents with minors with regard to a child's health information, the Privacy Rule states that state law governs. If a particular school receives specific funds from the U.S. Department of Education, then privacy protections are governed by the Family Educational Rights and Privacy Act of 1974 *(FERPA)* and the Protection of Pupil's Rights Amendment *(PPRA)*. For a full explanation, order the Guidelines for Protecting Confidential Student Health Information from www.ashaweb.org *(National Task Force on Confidential Studentl Health Information, 2000)*.

The Individuals with Disabilities Education Act (IDEA) deals with the appropriateness of releasing information about a student's disability which may or may not have bearing on issues related to reproductive health. For example, some states permit minors' access to contraceptive services and prenatal care without parental consent; others explicitly note a requirement for parental consent or parental notice *(The Alan Guttmacher Institute, 1997)*. It is important for school professionals to become familiar with their state laws, because they vary considerably. To find out about state laws school personnel can contact their state departments of education and health as well as the state attorney general's office.

It is critical that every school has a clear and appropriate policy. School personnel need to find out from their administrator or school board what written policy exists in their district regarding confidentiality related to issues such as sexual activity and pregnancy status. If none exists, they might suggest that one be established. Refer to *Guidelines for Protecting Confidential Student Health Information* published by the American School Health Association to inform the development process.

For more information about the Privacy Rule, contact the Office for Civil Rights Privacy web site at http://www.hhs.gov/ocr/hipaa/.
For information about FERPA, contact the U.S. Department of Education Family Compliance Office
400 Maryland Avenue, SW
Washington, DC 20202
(202) 260-3887

Record Keeping Tips

* School nurses, psychologists, social workers, and others should routinely keep all personal notes about students in locked files.

* Do not give confidential records to an unauthorized person to duplicate or file.

* Use standardized informed consent forms for permitting access to confidential information or disclosure of information.

* Consent forms themselves should be treated as confidential information because they often contain sensitive details.

* The outside of a folder of confidential information should list the names of people permitted to access it.

* Written permission for someone to access a file should specify the person's name, not position, so that a later person in the same position does not automatically have access.

—From Bogden, Fraser, Vega-Matos, & Ascroft. (1996). *Someone at School Has AIDS*.

Guidelines for Protecting Confidential Student Health Information, published by the American School Health Association (ASHA), gives guidance on protecting students' confidentiality while providing teachers and other school personnel with the health information they need to help students achieve their educational goals and maintain their health and safety and, at the same time, enabling health and mental health professionals to provide appropriate services. The guidelines are available from

ASHA, 7263 State Route 43/P.O. Box 708, Kent, OH 44240, http://www.ashaweb.org.

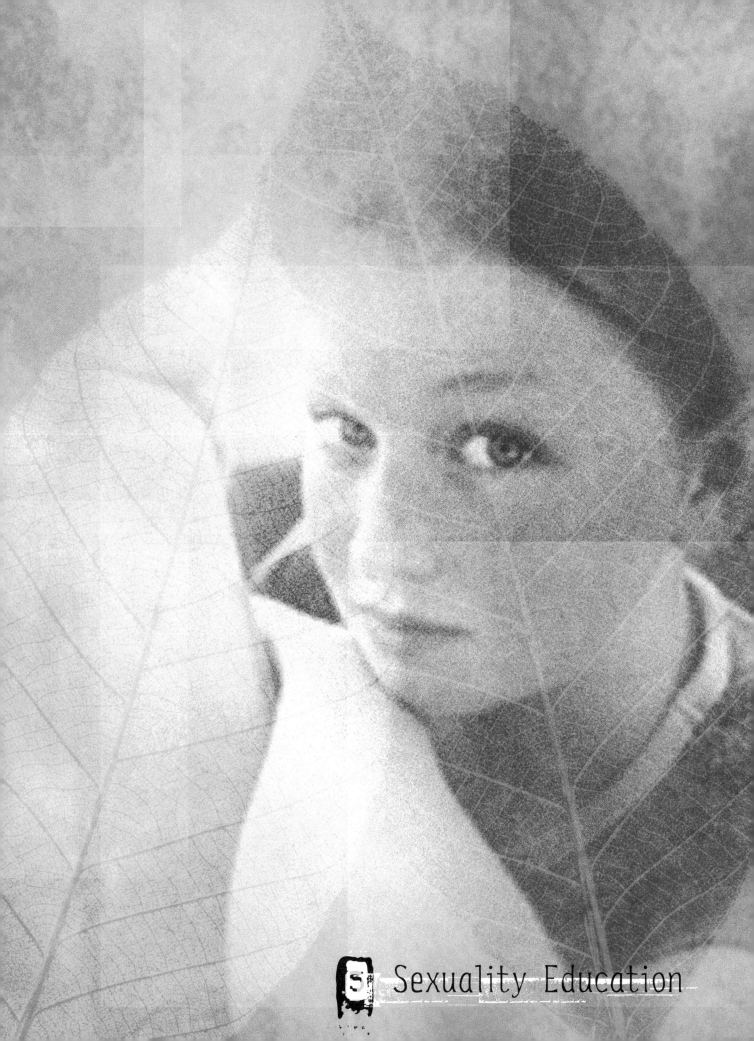

Sexuality Education

The Case For Sexuality Education

About 50 million children—95 percent of our nation's youth—attend public schools. Because they house virtually all of the nation's youth during their most developmentally critical years, schools play a fundamental role in helping students obtain answers to questions regarding their sexual health. As evidenced by several recent surveys, parents and students alike acknowledge the important role schools play in sexuality education. Students cite teachers and counselors as second only to their families in being trusted sources for sexuality-related information *(Kaiser Family Foundation, 2003)*. While few would disagree that parents should be their children's primary educators in this area, the fact is that many parents do not feel comfortable speaking with their children about issues related to sexual behavior. Parents who do talk with their children about puberty and sexuality do not always provide sufficient or accurate information. It is therefore not surprising that parents want schools teaching their children sexuality education. A majority of parents say they want their children to learn how to use condoms and birth control, as well as how to talk to their partners about sex. Approximately 93% of parents say that sex education programs in school have been helpful to their child in dealing with sexual issues. Three-quarters of parents want such

controversial topics as abortion and sexual orientation covered *(Kaiser Family Foundation, 2000a & 2003)*.

"Our laws can't keep up with the fact that kids are getting pregnant or sexually involved younger and younger. It is a Catch 22. Not all kids are ready for this in the 6th grade but what about those who are? That's when teachers, counselors, and nurses can reach these kids... as long as they can get parents' permission."
(Health Education Supervisor)

Students themselves report wanting more information about sexuality than their parents typically provide, including discussions about how to handle pressure to have sex and how to know when they are ready to become sexually active *(Kaiser Family Foundation, 2003)*. Unfortunately, there is a significant gap between what both students and parents want and what schools provide. This is important for two reasons. First, it indicates that students are not receiving the information that they need when it comes to sexuality education, and it shows the need for significant improvement on the part of parents and schools.

The Status of Sexuality Education in the Schools

Policy
District sexuality education policies govern program content, qualifications for teaching,

use of guest speakers, and parental permission for participation. Eighty-nine percent of all U.S. public school students will take sexuality education. Fifty-eight percent of principals report that their school has a comprehensive policy that treats abstinence as one option for adolescents in a broader sexuality program, 51% provide for teaching abstinence as the preferred option for adolescents but also permit discussion of contraception as an effective means of protecting against unintended pregnancy and disease, and 34% stipulate teaching abstinence as the only option outside of marriage, with discussion of contraception either prohibited entirely or permitted only to emphasize its deficiencies *(Kaiser Family Foundation, 2002)*.

Practice

The School Health Policies and Programs Study (SHPPS) conducted by the Centers for Disease Control and Prevention found that 57% of elementary schools, 76% of middle schools, and 82% of high schools surveyed required that human sexuality be taught. The teaching of pregnancy prevention was required in 19%, 55%, and 80% respectively, with HIV prevention education required in 50%, 76%, and 86% respectively and STD prevention in 25%, 69%, and 85% respectively *(Grunbaum et al., 2002)*. In a survey conducted by the Kaiser Family Foundation *(2000a)* 89% of students reported having had some form of sexuality education by grades 11-12.

Virtually all of the nation's nearly 20 million public secondary school students will take sexuality education at least once between 7th and 12th grades. Students report that the most frequently discussed topics are reproduction (90%) and abstinence (84%). Topics that are taught less frequently include using and obtaining birth control (59%), talking about birth control with a partner (58%), abortion (61%), rape and sexual assault (59%), and sexual orientation (41%). Areas that students want to know more about are: what to do in cases of rape or sexual assault, how to deal with the emotional consequences of being sexually active, how to talk with a partner about birth control and STDs, where to get and how to use birth control, and topics such as HIV/AIDS and other STDs *(Kaiser Family Foundation, 2000a)*.

Opinion

Public support for sexuality education is strong. Only 7% of Americans surveyed said that sex education should not be taught in schools. A national poll conducted in 2003 by NPR, the Kaiser Famiy Foundation, and Harvard University's Kennedy School of Government revealed that more than 90% of all Americans support the teaching of sexuality education in high school and just 15% who support sexuality education believe that sexuality education should be abstinence-only curricula *(Kaiser Family Foundation, 2003)*.

Principals in public schools report that the focus on abstinence-only instruction has increased from 2% in 1988 to 30% in 2003. Teachers say that, while topics such as HIV and STDs, abstinence, correct condom use, and resisting peer pressure are taught earlier than they were 10 years ago, most are taught less often and later than teachers think they should be. Ninety-three percent favor covering contraception; half believe it should be taught in grade seven or earlier. Yet one in four teachers are told not to teach the topic. One-third of teachers restricted what they taught because of concerns about adverse community reactions and one-fourth said the information they believed their students needed was not included in the curriculum they used *(The Alan Guttmacher Institute, 2000, Kaiser Family Foundation, 2003)*.

Types of Sexuality Education Programs

Despite inconsistencies in policy, practice, and opinion related to sexuality education, one thing that remains clear is the important role that schools play. With supportive programs and policies, schools can supplement and reinforce what students learn from their parents, while also countering the misinformation and mixed messages they are likely to get from the media and their friends. By discussing sexuality and reproduction openly, teens learn to accept these as normal parts of the life cycle but ones that require serious thought and responsibility *(National Guidelines Task Force, 1996)*. A variety of programs exist, differing in a number of ways, but primarily in how they address the topic of contraception:

* **Abstinence-only** education and abstinence-until-marriage programs present abstinence as the only 100% protection against unplanned pregnancy, HIV, and STDs. The abstinence-only philosophy assumes that teenagers should postpone sexual intercourse until they are adults. Abstinence-until-marriage programs promote the idea that teens should postpone sexual intercourse until they are married. These programs either do not include discussion about contraceptive options or discuss the failure of contraceptives to provide complete protection *(Kirby, 1997)*.

* **Abstinence-based** programs present abstinence as the best option for teens whether or not they have been sexually active in the past. They help teens build the skills to choose abstinence until they are emotionally and physically mature, and to understand options for contraceptive use when they decide to become sexually active *(Kirby, 2001)*.

* **Comprehensive sexuality education** programs view sexuality education as a lifelong process and address sexual development, reproductive health, interpersonal relationships, affection, intimacy, body image, gender roles, abstinence, and contraceptive options *(National Guidelines Task Force, 1996)*.

* **Family life education** programs engage students in the development of plans for careers, marriage, family life, and budgeting.

Which Approach Is Best

Abstinence from sexual intercourse is the only 100% sure way to avoid pregnancy. For students who choose to engage in sexual behavior, consistent and correct use of contraception can significantly reduce the risk for unintended pregnancy, HIV and other STDs. Advocates for abstinence-only programs claim that comprehensive sexuality programs give students a mixed message, by warning them to avoid sex while at the same time providing them with the skills to use condoms should they become sexually active. But the research discounts this notion. Evaluations have shown that comprehensive sexuality programs do not increase the onset of intercourse and that, in fact, some have delayed the onset of intercourse or have increased condom use among sexually active youth. To date no studies have found any consistent or significant effects of abstinence-only programs upon delaying the onset of intercourse, yet little rigorous evaluation of abstinence-only programs has been completed. Evidence of the effectiveness of abstinence-only programs is not yet conclusive (*Kirby, 2001*).

The U.S. Department of Health and Human Services has contracted with Mathematica Policy Research, Inc., to evaluate abstinence education programs funded by Title V of the Social Security Act. The evaluation asks the question "To what extent are abstinence education programs effective in persuading youth to be sexually abstinent and in changing teen sexual behavior?" (*Devaneyat et al., 2002*). An interim report is available on Mathematica's website: *http://www.mathematica-mpr.com*.

Research has clearly shown that the most effective school-based programs are comprehensive ones that include a focus on both abstinence and condom use (*Kirby, 2001*). Debra Hafner, former president of SIECUS, points out that young people can handle mixed messages about sex in the same way that they handle messages about drinking and driving—"We tell teenagers not to drink, but we also warn them that if they do drink, they shouldn't drive" (*Black, 1998*).

A research panel commissioned by the National Campaign to Prevent Teen Pregnancy found the following nine characteristics common to programs that have been proven effective in educating youth to adopt sexual risk reduction behaviors (*Kirby, 2001*):

* Focus clearly on reducing one or more sexual behaviors that can lead to unintended pregnancy or HIV/STD infection.

* Incorporate behavioral goals, teaching methods, and materials that are appropriate to the age, sexual experience, and culture of the students.

* Are based on theoretical approaches that have been demonstrated to be effective in

Title V

Title V, Section 510 of the Social Security Act, authorized under the Personal Responsibility and Work Opportunity Reconciliation Act of 1996, includes funding for state abstinence education programs. Abstinence education programs funded through this grant program must teach an unambiguous abstinence message to youth and may not provide instruction in the use of birth control or to promote the use of such methods. This funding is administered by the Administration for Children, Youth, and Families. The governor of each state determines which agency will administer the Section 510 program statewide. Since the 1996 law, additional federal funding has been allocated to abstinence education programming. In an amendment to a fiscal year (FY) 2000 omnibus spending bill, Congress approved $20 million for abstinence-only education through the Title V Block Grant's Special Projects of Regional and National Significance (SPRANS).

A program receiving this funding must:

* Have as its exclusive purpose teaching the social, psychological, and health gains to be realized by abstaining from sexual activity

* Teach abstinence from sexual activity outside marriage as the expected standard for all school-age children

* Teach that abstinence from sexual activity is the only certain way to avoid out-of-wedlock pregnancy, sexually transmitted diseases, and other associated health problems

* Teach that a mutually faithful, monogamous relationship in the context of marriage is the expected standard of sexual activity

* Teach that sexual activity outside the context of marriage is likely to have harmful psychological and physical effects

* Teach that bearing children out-of-wedlock is likely to have harmful consequences for the child, the child's parents, and society

* Teach young people how to reject sexual advances and how alcohol and drug use increases vulnerability to sexual advances

* Teach the importance of attaining self-sufficiency before engaging in sexual activity

Grant guidelines state that "It is not necessary to place equal emphasis on each element of the definition. However, a project may not be inconsistent with any aspect of the abstinence education definition." For the current grant guidelines, visit http://www.acf.hhs.gov/programs/fysb/absfund-anncmt.htm

Implementation varies greatly among states, ranging from brief, curriculum-based classroom programs to more intensive ones with many complementary services or "boosters" to reinforce the abstinence messages and to provide youth with alternatives to high-risk

after-school care, tutoring and other forms of academic support, peer or adult mentors, motivational assemblies, cultural events, and parent and family support and education programs. Many states have encouraged and supported community-wide abstinence ini-

tiatives, which attempt to alter behaviors through a combination of targeted services to youth and efforts to create systemic changes in community norms, messages, and support (Devaney et al., 2002).

influencing other health-related risks.

* Deliver and consistently reinforce a clear message about abstaining from sexual activity and/or using condoms or other forms of contraception.

* Last long enough to allow participants to complete important activities.

* Provide basic, accurate information about the risks of unprotected inter-course and methods of avoiding unpro-tected intercourse.

* Employ a variety of teaching methods designed to involve the participants and help them personalize the information.

* Include activities that address social pressures related to sex.

* Provide modeling and practice in commu-nication, negotiation, and refusal skills.

* Select teachers or peers who believe in the program and then provide them with training, which often includes practice sessions.

Skill-building is key, no matter what approach a district chooses. To manage abstinent behavior, students need to be able

to avoid situations where they might be tempted to have sex, be capable of clearly communicating to another person their desire to be abstinent, and know how to effec-tively resist pressure not to remain abstinent. To manage having sex safely, students need skills to obtain and use protection effec-tively and to communicate with and gain the support and cooperation of their partner for carrying out protective behaviors.

Evaluated Programs

A number of curricula have shown evidence of effectively reducing sexual risk behaviors that contribute to HIV and STD infection and unintended pregnancy.

Reducing the Risk: Building Skills to Prevent Pregnancy, HIV, and STD (RTR) targets students in grades 9-10. The curriculum emphasizes avoiding unprotected intercourse by practicing abstinence or by using contra-ception. Through role plays, participants learn to recognize and resist peer pressure, make decisions, and negotiate safe sexual behaviors. Students are encouraged to talk to their parents about abstinence and birth control and to visit stores and clinics to learn more about birth control. The curriculum consists of a teacher's manual, a student workbook (available in English or Spanish), and an activity kit. For ordering or training information contact *ETR Associates, P.O. Box 1830; Santa Cruz, CA 95061; (800) 321-4407; http://www.etr.org.*

Becoming a Responsible Teen (BART) is an HIV intervention developed for 14-18 year-old African-American youth. Designed to be offered in a non-academic, community-based setting and facilitated by a male and a female group leader in gender-specific groups, the curriculum addresses risk reduction, communication, negotiation, refusal skills, problem solving, and condom use through interactive sessions that include games, role plays, and videos. It has proven to be effective with both sexually-experienced and sexually-abstinent youth. For ordering or training information contact *ETR Associates, P.O. Box 1830; Santa Cruz, CA 95061; (800) 321-4407; http://www.etr.org.*

Safer Choices, a two-year HIV, STD, and pregnancy prevention curriculum for grades 9-10, integrates a classroom curriculum with school-wide activities including a health promotion council, peer teams, parent involvement, staff development, and community linkages. The components of this program include levels 1 and 2 curricula, a peer leaders' guide, an implementation manual, and an activity kit. For ordering or training information contact *ETR Associates, P.O. Box 1830; Santa Cruz, CA 95061;*

(800) 321-4407; http://www.etr.org.

Be Proud! Be Responsible! focuses on AIDS prevention by aiming to improve AIDS-related knowledge and attitudes among male adolescents in urban environments. Through group discussion, participants learn the risks of injected drug use and unsafe sexual behaviors. Videos, role plays, games, and exercises reinforce learning and encourage participation. The curriculum and video can be ordered through *Select Media, Inc., 18 Harrison Street, 5th Floor, New York, NY 10013; (800) 707-6334.* For information on training contact *ETR Associates, P.O. Box 1830, Santa Cruz, CA 95061; (800) 321-4407; http://www.etr.org*

Get Real About AIDS, designed for grades 9-12, is an HIV prevention curriculum that addresses sexual risk-taking behaviors related to teen pregnancy prevention. To order, contact *AGC United Learning; 1560 Sherman Avenue, Suite 100, Evanston, IL 60201; (800) 323-9084; www.unitedlearning.com.* For information about training, call the *Comprehensive Health Education Foundation, (800) 323-CHEF.*

For a partial listing of other promising sexuality education programs, refer to the resources section at the end of this chapter. Use the following questions to help select the most appropriate curricula for your school.

Questions to Ask When Selecting a Sexuality Education Curriculum

✳ Is the curriculum research-based? Is the content scientifically accurate, i.e., does research support statements offered as facts? What are the credentials of the developers?

✳ Is there provision for adequate staff training, including accurate information, self-examination of personal attitudes, and skill building?

✳ Does the curriculum address only sexual intercourse or the broad spectrum of sexuality, including relationships, communication, and respect?

✳ Does the curriculum help students acquire skills to abstain from sexual activity and receive accurate, comprehensive information about contraception?

✳ Is the curriculum age-appropriate and does it avoid stereotypes and biases?

✳ Does the curriculum include parents and guardians as partners with the schools?

—Adapted from Wiley and Terlosky, 2000.

Incorporating Teen Pregnancy Prevention Education Across Curricula

In U.S. public secondary schools, more than half of those delivering sexuality education are teachers of health education or physical education. But in some schools this responsibility is shared by a variety of professionals. For instance, biology and consumer science teachers account for one-fifth of those delivering sexuality education in public secondary schools, and school nurses make up 3% *(Darroch, Landry, & Singh, 2000)*. At the elementary level, classroom teachers constitute more than three-quarters of sexuality education teachers with nurses (13%) and physical or health education and science teachers delivering the rest (10%) *(Landry, Singh, & Darroch, 2000)*.

Sexuality education is often delivered as one of many lessons given within a semester. It is important to note that one of the nine characteristics of effective sexuality education curricula is that they last long enough to cover all of the important skills-building activities. *Reducing the Risk*, for example, requires 17 class periods. At the same time, teachers and schools are under pressure to keep their students up to par academically. Consequently, sexuality education lessons are often condensed and squeezed into the already full lesson plan. Teachers need to be creative with the time that they do have to infuse critical sexuality and health education messages into other lessons. To supplement and reinforce health education and human development lessons, teachers of other topics can incorporate relevant messages without deviating from their own teaching objectives. For example:

- In math class, compare the incidence of teen pregnancy or STD/AIDS in the county to that of the state and the nation.

- In civics or economics classes, pose the question "How do you think teen pregnancy affects the community?"

- In English class, use descriptions of relationships and gender roles described in poetry and literature to discuss social pressures and communication skills.

- In journalism class or classes addressing current events, examine stereotyping or the unrealistic portrayal of consequences in the media.

- In social studies, use current events to discuss healthy and unhealthy decision-making.

- In geography, discuss the disparate impact of AIDS on particular regions of the world.

- In family and consumer sciences explore the implications of becoming a parent, including parenting education, weekly expenses for sustaining a family, balancing a budget, and identifying appropriate living space.

For easy-to-use fact sheets with statistics on a wide variety of adolescent health topics, visit Advocates for Youth's web site at *http://www.advocatesforyouth.org*.

Other Promising Programs

Sex Can Wait: An Abstinence Program for grades 5-12 allows students to focus on abstinence as the safest choice. The curriculum aims to build student knowledge and skills before they become involved in sexual relationships. Available from *ETR Associates, Phone: (800) 321-4407, Fax: (800) 435-8433, Website: http://www.etr.org*.

Postponing Sexual Involvement (PSI) uses older teens, educators, nurses, and counselors to stress the importance of sexual abstinence among younger teens. PSI teaches decision making and negotiation skills, using role play to help students recognize and develop responses to peer pressure. It stresses abstinence but incorporates contraceptive information and decision-making skills.

Postponing Sexual Involvement: Young Teens and *Postponing Sexual Involvement: Preteens* are available from *The Center for Adolescent Reproductive Health, Box 26158 —Emory/Grady Teen Services Program, Grady Memorial Hospital, 80 Butler St., S.E., Atlanta, GA 30330-3801 (404) 616-3513*.

Life Planning Education, appropriate for youth ages 13-18, provides interactive exercises, handouts, and a guide for implementation to address skill-building, values, self-esteem, relationships, parenthood, employment preparation, and reducing sexual risk. Available for $75 (400-page loose-leaf binder) from Advocates for Youth *1025 Vermont Avenue, N.W., Suite 200, Washington, DC 20005 Phone: (202) 347-5700 Website: http://www.advocatesforyouth.org*

Resources

▶ *Guidelines for Comprehensive Sexuality Education: Kindergarten—12th Grade* is organized by four developmental levels (early elementary, late elementary, middle school, high school) with 36 topics addressed within six main concepts— human development, relationships, personal skills, sexual behavior, sexual health, and society and culture.

Developed by a national task force of health, education, and sexuality professionals to help communities design new curricula or assess and revise existing ones the document is available from SIECUS (Sexuality Information and Education Council of the U.S.), 130 W. 42nd Street, Suite 350, New York, NY 10036. Phone: (212) 819-9770. **Website:** http://www.siecus.org

▶ *The Sexuality Education Challenge: Promoting Healthy Sexuality in Young People*, edited by Judy C. Drolet and Kay Clark, examines issues including sexuality education in schools, teacher preparation, diversity, community programs and partnerships, and evaluation and research. The book is available from ETR Associates, P.O. Box 1830, Santa Cruz, CA 95061-1830 Phone: (800) 321-4407. **Website:** http://www.etr.org

▶ *Resource Center for Adolescent Pregnancy Prevention (RECAPP)*, a website maintained by ETR Associates (http://www.etr.org/recapp) provides regularly updated information on programs and resources.

▶ *Abstinence the Better Choice, Inc.* offers training on the Responsible Social Values Program for educators who wish to provide abstinence until marriage education at the middle school level. *Training for Concerned About Teen Sexuality (C.A.T.S.)* is available to adult leadership and high school students who wish to become members of C.A.T.S. For information contact:
Abstinence the Better Choice, Inc.
1815 W. Market St., Ste. 110
Akron, OH 44313
Phone: (330) 864-1359
Website: http://www.abstinencebetter-choice.com

Sample Lesson Plan

A school counselor in an Iowa middle school was concerned about the numbers of girls who were coming to her for help with decisions about relationships. When she found out that her county had the highest rate of STDs in the state, she asked the school board for permission to start a prevention program at the middle school. Students are either invited by the counselor or volunteer for small groups conducted in her office. She combines lessons from *Reducing the Risk* with *It Takes Two* which focuses on relationships. Below is a lesson plan outline.

Learning Objectives:

Students will be able to:

* Evaluate risks and consequences of becoming an adolescent parent or becoming infected with HIV or another STD

* Recognize that abstaining from sexual activity is the only 100 percent effective way to avoid pregnancy, HIV infection, and other STDs

* Learn that using protection can help to avoid pregnancy, HIV infection, and other STDs

* Demonstrate effective communication skills for remaining abstinent and avoiding unprotected sexual intercourse

* Understand the difference between a healthy and an unhealthy relationship

Sessions

1. *Relationships: The Search for Love.* Discussion of the roles of self-esteem and acceptance in a healthy relationship. An introduction to facts about teen pregnancy.

2. *Living in Relationships.* A discussion of what makes a healthy relationship, power issues, and dating violence.

3. *Abstinence, Sex, and Protection.* Refusal skills and an activity to demonstrate vulnerability to pregnancy.

4. *Abstinence.* Discussion of the advantages of abstinence, reasons teens fail to abstain or use protection, and elements of successful communication about abstinence.

5. *Refusals.* Discussion of characteristics of effective refusals and role play. An assignment in which students talk to their parents about sex.

6. *Using Refusal Skills.* More practice.

7. *Avoiding High-Risk Situations.* Discuss and practice managing situations that can lead to unwanted or unprotected sex. Myths and truths about protection from pregnancy and STDs.

Continued on next page.

Continued from page 42.

8. **Protection: Myths and Truths.** Review discussion of abstinence, condoms, and spermicides—how each method works and its reliability.

9. **Skills Integration.** Additional opportunities to practice decision-making and refusal skills, using scripted situations in which students decide as a group how to handle difficult situations.

10. **Preventing HIV and Other STDs.** Exploration of five specific STDs (genital warts, gonorrhea, herpes, chlamydia, HIV)—symptoms, transmission, and prevention, ending with an exercise on how HIV would change their lives.

11. **Skills Integration.** The importance of sticking with choices.

(Adapted from South Tama County, Iowa)

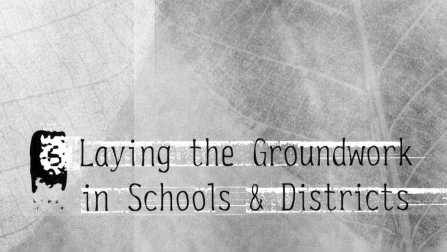
Laying the Groundwork
in Schools & Districts

Assessing the Status of Pregnancy Prevention in A School or District

Before making a proposal for teen pregnancy prevention activities, school personnel need to find out what is already happening in their school, district, and community. For example, does the school district have a policy to teach sexuality education? More than two-thirds of school districts do. The remaining third leave the decision up to individual schools *(Kaiser Family Foundation, 2000)*. Does the district

What Is my School or District Doing to Prevent Teen Pregnancy and Promote Responsible Sexual Behavior?

Does my school or district have policies that address sexuality education, sexual harassment, and pregnant and parenting teens? What are they?

Is there a teen pregnancy prevention committee or a health advisory committee? Who is on the committee? What financial and personnel support does the committee have? What is the relationship between the health advisory committee and the school improvement committee?

Has a needs assessment been conducted? What are the findings?

What type of sexuality education is being provided and by whom? Are curricula research-based and have they been evaluated and found to be effective?

Have teachers been trained to teach the curricula? How much of the curricula is actually being taught?

How many students are being reached and in which grades? Have students had the opportunity to provide feedback regarding how well sexuality education programs are meeting their needs?

What reproductive health counseling and services are available for young people?

What programs and services are available for pregnant and parenting teens?

Who on staff has been trained on teen pregnancy prevention policies and programs and the roles that each staff member can play?

How are families involved in school or district teen pregnancy prevention activities? What opportunities have been offered to inform and involve families? How much family participation is there? What are barriers and supports to family involvement in your school or district?

What teen pregnancy prevention programs exist in the community? (Use Chart 1 in appendix B). How does the district or the school cooperate with community pregnancy prevention programs and youth development activities?

have school-based or school-linked health centers? If so, do they provide reproductive health services? About half of school-based health centers serving middle and high schools offer reproductive health services, including family planning services, pregnancy testing, treatment for STDs, and HIV/AIDS counseling though the majority do not dispense contraception *(NASBHC, 2002)*. The questions on page 53 can help to determine what is in place and apply that information to set goals and objectives to fill existing gaps. Chart I: *Inventory of School and Community Programs, Activities, and Policies to Prevent Teen Pregnancy* (Appendix B, page 148) is designed to help map what currently exists in a school or district.

Considerations for Developing a Plan to Promote Responsible Sexual Behavior

* **What are we proposing? Is there research to support it? Have we developed a strong case for our proposal?**

* **What state and local policies exist? How do they support this proposal? Do local policies need to be reassessed and updated? Are there sample policies that can serve as a model?**

* **What data will support the need for a teen pregnancy prevention program?** (teen pregnancy rate, teen birthrate, HIV and other STD infection rate, incidence of sexual abuse, sexual harassment, and dating violence)

* **Where can these data be found?** state, county, and local health departments; hospitals and clinics; school nurse or health center and other school health and mental health records; police departments; social service agencies; state departments of education

* **Who are my allies?** school administrators, parents, students, teachers, other school staff, NEA affiliates, youth-serving agencies, religious leaders, business community

* **How does what we are proposing relate to other activities we have identified in the community?** (What Is My School Or District Doing To Prevent Teen Pregnancy and Promote Sexually Responsible Behavior?)

* **Do we have a plan?**

* **Are our objectives realistic?**

* **How do we propose to fund or otherwise support this proposal?**

* **How will we know that what we are doing is working? How will we evaluate what we have done?**

Obtaining Administrative Support

No program or policy can succeed without the support of school administrators and policymakers. The school board is charged with setting education policy and giving direction to the superintendent. Policy development should include teachers, administrators, other school staff, community organizations, businesses, families, students, the faith community, and other concerned citizens. If the district does not already have a policy on teen pregnancy prevention, this is a logical place to begin. If a policy exists, the district needs to determine whether it needs to be updated to reflect current state policy and the latest research. If the district is planning to introduce a new curriculum or after-school activity, it needs to determine how it fits with existing school policies.

Before going to the school board, proponents will need to obtain the understanding and support of the superintendent, the principal, the curriculum coordinator, and the director of student support services, all of whom will be affected by what is being proposed. Proponents might also wish to consult with the school health advisory committee, if one exists. At these preliminary meetings proponents need to review the proposal and present the data they plan to present to the school board. The message should highlight the link between pregnancy prevention and academic achievement and how this effort relates to the work of the school improvement team, if one exists. Proponents need to firmly advocate for their message, but also be prepared to listen. When hearing the rationale for the proposal, advisors might offer suggestions for strengthening the approach.

How to Prepare A Presentation for Policymakers

✳ Familiarize yourself with your state and district policies. Find out what other laws and regulations (local, state, and federal) apply to what you are proposing.

NARAL Pro Choice America has published Who Decides? A State by State Review of Abortion and Reproductive Rights, which provides information about each state's laws regarding sexuality and STD/HIV education.

Some states require schools to provide sexuality education. Of those states, a few require sexuality education but not the inclusion of information about contraception. Others require that sexuality education teach abstinence and provide information about contraception. Most states require schools to provide STD, HIV, and/or AIDS education. Many of those states require that STD, HIV, and/or AIDS education programs teach abstinence and other methods of prevention. States which do not require sexuality education may still make recommendations or set guidelines for what is taught if a district chooses to provide STD, HIV/AIDS, and/or pregnancy prevention. Many also address requirements for parental consent, which range from written permission for participation in a course to written parental request to excuse students from participation (NARAL 2005 (http:www.prochoiceameri-ca.org/ yourstate/whodecides/index.cfm).

Information about your state's school health education policies are available from your state department of education.

✳ Gather local and state data to support the need for teen pregnancy prevention.

LOCAL SOURCES

Your local health department can provide data such as incidence of teen pregnancy, teen birth rates, and incidence of STDs. School nurses can provide anecdotal information and data such as the number and kinds of problems for which students visit their office and the number of referrals for pregnancy and STDs. Hospital records and social service agencies have data on admissions related to reproductive health and instances of abuse. Police departments should have data on incidences of sexual violence.

STATE SOURCES

The state department of health, especially the maternal and child health division, and the state office of vital statistics can provide statistics on teen pregnancy. The state department of education in most states conducts the Youth Risk Behavior Survey (YRBS) which gathers data on the proportion of high school students in the state who engage in sexual behaviors that put them at risk for pregnancy. Sometimes YRBS data are available for individual communities. Some communities use the YRBS survey protocol to gather local data for themselves. To learn more about the YRBS go to the CDC's Division of Adolescent and School Health website (http://www.cdc.gov/HealthyYouth). Another state-by-state data source is Kids Count (http://www.aecf.org/kidscount). The National Campaign to Prevent Teen Pregnancy website (http://www.teenpregnancy.org) has teen birth rates for many counties.

* Recruit allies. (See Chapter 8, Building Community Support.) Find others in your school or community who are concerned about teen pregnancy and are willing to support this effort. These include parents, teachers, clergy, health and mental health professionals, business people, representatives of your NEA affiliate, youth-serving organizations, and other community agencies. If you are relatively new to the district, you may find it helpful to identify an ally who is a long-time resident, well-known, and trusted by policymakers. Several people interviewed for this publication mentioned that they found obtaining approval relatively easy because the school community knew them or an advocate with whom they collaborated trusted them.

Don't overlook student involvement. Schools tend to be supportive of student-initiated activities (Washington State, 1999). Students know what is happening in their school community, can be convincing proponents, and can rally their peers. And if they exist in your community, school improvement committees and district or community health advisory councils can be critical players.

* Make a strong case for the role of schools in pregnancy prevention. Point out the links between academic outcomes and involvement in risky behaviors. Adolescent health data suggest that students who feel valued, whose teachers and families have high expectations, and who have strong connection to families and schools are less likely to be involved in risky behaviors. The American School Health Association has developed an advocacy kit that can be a helpful resource for preparing this type of presentation.

* Propose a plan. Create realistic objectives and suggest activities to meet those objectives. Cite research to support the effectiveness of what you are proposing. One successful advocate in Iowa prepared a packet that included local data on STDs and student self-reported behaviors compared to statewide and national data, a curriculum outline, a sample parent permission letter, and a timeline for implementation.

Sample Script for a School Board Presentation

We appreciate your placing this item on this evening's agenda. The proposal we are bringing to the board today recommends that the .... district expand the curriculum at the middle school to address a growing concern about adolescent risk for pregnancy, HIV, and other STDs. The name of the curriculum/program we are suggesting is .... In keeping with this district's policies, the program's major focus is abstinence and the practice of communication skills to prevent pregnancy and the transmission of STDs. The program is based upon research and has been evaluated in communities similar to ours. Evaluation results demonstrated positive behavior changes among students participating in the program.

School counselors, nurses, and teachers who work directly with students overwhelmingly feel that pregnancy and sexually transmitted disease prevention among the youth of our community needs to be addressed by the schools. Teen parenthood is the leading cause of high school dropout for young women. Because it threatens the academic achievement of students, teen pregnancy is an issue we cannot ignore. This proposal is based on the combined recommendations of members of the School Health Advisory Committee and the School Improvement Committee.

(Provide and review handouts with data that demonstrate the numbers or percentages of adolescents with STDs, AIDS cases, and live births to teens in the county; a description of the proposed program; endorsements from members of the community; and a proposed timeline for implementation.)

We conducted a survey in (month) on local middle school students' attitudes and behaviors and compared the findings with youth nationally and at the state level. Students were asked whether they had ever had sexual intercourse, and, if so, whether they were protecting themselves with a condom. ....% of .... graders reported having had intercourse at least once. Of those students........% reported always using contraceptives. You will note that the percentage of sexually active students is higher than the national norm and that our county ranks among the highest in the state.

This information provided by professionals working directly with the students, by the department of public health, and by the students themselves strongly indicates the importance of addressing the subject of pregnancy and disease prevention. The handouts we have given you include summaries of these findings, a description of the proposed program, letters of support from members of the community, a proposed timeline for implementation, and an estimate of resources required. Please note that among our first activities will be a parent and community awareness meeting at which we will describe the program, invite questions, and respond to concerns.

Do you have any questions for us? Thank you for your time. We hope that you will support the introduction of this program.

A Sample Timeline for Obtaining Support

OCTOBER

School Health Advisory Committee (SHAC) meets to discuss growing number of younger students involved with risky behaviors.

NOVEMBER - DECEMBER

SHAC members conduct an inventory of current district efforts
(See page 45 "What Is My School or District Doing To Prevent Teen Pregnancy and Promote Responsible Sexual Behavior?").

DECEMBER - JANUARY

SHAC meets to identify gaps.

SHAC researches program options.

FEBRUARY - MARCH

SHAC presents options to the school improvement committee, school nurses, counselors, psychologists, district superintendent, curriculum coordinator, school principals, and the county nurse.

APRIL - MAY

SHAC designees agree to write a proposal, take it to the school board, and get parent input.

Proposal is presented to school board.

Letters are sent to parents, explaining the program and inviting input.

JUNE

A second meeting is scheduled with the school board to obtain feedback and report parent reaction.

If school board and parent input are positive, SHAC begins plans to initiate the program during next school year.

Preparing School Staff to Support Pregnancy Prevention Activities

Most health educators, counselors, and nurses are professionally trained to deal with the sensitive issues associated with children's and adolescents' developing sexuality, but may need additional training to get comfortable. Moreover, sexuality education is often taught by classroom teachers. In grades 5 and 6, 77% of sexuality education teachers are classroom teachers, while 13% are school nurses and 10% are physical or health education or science teachers *(Landry et al., 2000)*. While four out of five sexuality education teachers report having had training to teach the topic *(Kaiser, 2000)*, 40-53% of grades 5 and 6 sexuality education teachers report needing some kind of assistance—teaching materials, strategies, or factual information *(Landry et al., 2000)*.

Many teachers also cite pressures from parents, the community, and the school administration related to sexuality education. Forty-six percent said that such pressures are one of their three biggest problems *(Landry et al., 2000)*. The school district needs to provide training for all district personnel to increase their comfort and skill level both with the subject matter and the pressures they feel. However, teachers should not be required to teach sexuality education if they continue to feel uncomfortable with the topic. The district training should ensure that they can:

* understand district policies related to risk behaviors and confidentiality

* be familiar with concepts taught in the classroom so that they can reinforce this learning in their contacts with students

* be aware of resources in the school and the community where students might get help

* know to whom to speak should they have a question or become aware of a student's need for referral to a community resource

* understand what constitutes developmentally appropriate information and behavior and how to present it

* be comfortable with and understand their own values relating to sexuality

Offering this training to all district personnel can help to ensure that students receive a consistent message and staff will know how to respond appropriately to actions or words that cause concern. Some training topics, such as district pregnancy prevention plans, activities, and policies; data about teen pregnancy and other risk behaviors in the community; and school and community resources, will be applicable to all school personnel. Other aspects will be specific to the staff persons' particular roles within the district and will need to be tailored to their special concerns. Training should provide opportunities to observe modeling and practice skills. After the entire staff has been trained, training can be offered to new staff annually as they join the district. As new data, programs, and resources emerge, schedule training to reinforce and update previous information. Who conducts the training depends on the district's size, capacity and the kind of training desired. Trainers—either district employees or outside consultants—can be health education, mental health, or health professionals with expertise in areas of reproductive health and youth development.

Questions for Planning Staff Training

※ Who is responsible for planning the training? Who will help?

※ How will we find out what staff already know? How will we find out what they want or need to learn more about? (Needs Assessment)

※ Who will provide the training?

※ What will be the content and design? Will there be opportunities for skill building as well as receiving information? How will we address sensitive issues?

※ When and where will the training occur?

※ How will we ensure participation? How will we promote the training?

※ Will the superintendent, principal, or school board members be there to demonstrate support? How much time will we need?

※ What resources will be needed, (e.g., release time, trainer stipends, handouts, refreshments) and how will we pay for them?

※ How will we follow up and reinforce what staff have learned?

Worksheet for Planning Staff Training/Orientation

GOAL: **To prepare school personnel to support teen pregnancy prevention and other student health promotion activities**

TARGET AUDIENCE: **All school personnel**

PROPOSED OBJECTIVES:

* **Introduce the purpose of the training**

  1) To ensure that staff give students a consistent message.

  2) To prepare staff to:

     * provide students with accurate, age-appropriate information

     * help students develop and build upon personal strengths

     * respond appropriately to student actions or words that cause concern

* **Explain why teen pregnancy prevention and other activities to promote sexual responsibility are needed in the district or school.**

  1) The extent of teen pregnancy and other sexual behaviors in the community

  2) How this compares to state and national data

* **Inform school personnel regarding district policies related to teen pregnancy prevention and other activities to promote sexual responsibility.**

  Examples might include: abstinence-only and abstinence-based sexuality education; a safe environment (sexual harassment, sexual orientation); pregnant and parenting teens; family and community involvement; requirements for staff training, etc.

* **Present district programs designed to implement policies and address specific issues.**

  Examples might include sexuality education curricula; peer education activities; coordinated school health program; school-based health centers; condom availability; mentoring; etc.

* **Discuss how school personnel can support these activities.**

  Learn about the programs; volunteer to participate; incorporate activities into courses; be alert for warning signs of risk behaviors; be prepared to respond or intervene as appropriate; promote a respectful positive school climate.

* **Discuss special concerns:**

  1) How to address sensitive issues such as abortion, sexual orientation, condoms, masturbation, sexual harassment, dating violence, etc.

  2) Confidentiality and how to respond when a student confides or behaves in a way that causes concern.

  3) Developmentally appropriate behavior and providing age-appropriate information.

  4) Working with students with special needs.

  5) Communicating with parents and other community members.

* **Include exercises to explore school personnel's values, feelings, and attitudes toward sexuality and to strengthen their comfort with the topic**

* Provide information about resources available to support school personnel in efforts to prevent teen pregnancy and promote sexually responsible behavior.
  1) Where to find answers to questions (people, agencies, print documents, websites)
  2) Who in the school or district is conducting programs and how they can help
  3) Referral procedures

* Prepare school personnel to fulfill their role, e.g., model behaviors, practice skill building.

* Offer plans for follow-up and reinforcement.

* Invite participants to evaluate training and offer suggestions for future staff development.

Maintaining Administrative Support

Addressing sensitive topics such as those related to sexuality education requires the continued support of the administration and the community. Below are some tips for doing so.

* Keep policymakers fully informed about activities and any changes in implementation.

* Update students, school staff, and families regularly with activities such as publishing a newsletter or providing articles to the school newspaper. Provide opportunities for feedback. Share and respond to feedback.

* Coordinate activities. Communicate with other school and community agency staff who can support and reinforce the program and cooperate to expand activities. Be on the look out for opportunities to create linkages. One school health coordinator lamented that in her district some teachers are teaching reproductive health, school nurses go to some classrooms, and home economics teachers teach family life but nobody knows who is doing what. As she put it, "I don't even know how many kids are pregnant. The district may have the data but, since we don't collaborate, health services may have it—they may be doing something that health education doesn't even know about." This situation could be avoided with open communication and collaboration among staff.

* Gather data which includes positive feedback from students and parents to show that the program is well-received.

An Idea from the Field

A school nurse in Mississippi puts materials in the display case near the principal's office. Because everybody goes by there, they notice and look at them.

State standards testing requirements often determine classroom teaching content. As a result, when requirements do not include sexuality education and other health-related topics, many districts are reluctant to make room in a full curriculum for these topics.

The New Jersey State Board of Education has adopted a standard that "all students will learn the physical, emotional and social aspects of human relationships and sexuality and apply these concepts to support a healthy, active lifestyle. Visit http:www.state.nj.us/njded/aps/cccs/chpe/faq.htm for the complete policy.

One County's Human Growth and Development Program

The Polk County, Florida School District, with 112 schools and about 80,000 students, has a comprehensive K-12 human growth and development program. Fundamental components of this program are:

* an appropriate and carefully designed curriculum for the appropriate grades
* well-qualified and trained teachers
* parental involvement
* strong administrative leadership
* a consistent philosophy on human sexuality throughout the school district

The program is intended to support and strengthen the role of family, community, religious, and other institutions in promoting healthy physical, emotional, and moral development by:

* encouraging responsible decision-making about sexual behavior
* building a healthy attitude toward all parts of the body and developing confidence and pride in being a male or female
* developing the life management skills needed to become a healthy, responsible, and self-disciplined adult
* facilitating community partnerships to reinforce program goals

CURRICULUM OVERVIEW

The K-12 human growth and development curriculum begins in kindergarten by including in lessons about germs the message that HIV is not spread by casual contact. In Grades 4 and 5 a registered nurse teaches lessons on puberty and the reproductive system. The middle school curriculum covers topics such as healthy relationships, dating behaviors, problems associated with early sexual involvement, date rape, and consequences of teen pregnancy. High school courses build on these themes, emphasizing the importance of marriage and planned pregnancies for the most desirable outcomes for mothers and their babies. Methods of contraception are discussed in the context of marriage and family planning. Abstinence is presented as the healthiest pregnancy prevention choice for unmarried adolescents. Issues addressed in Grades 11 and 12 include marriage, responsibilities of parenthood, genetics, fertility, and sound decision-making.

ADDRESSING CRITICAL ISSUES

The Polk County Public Schools comprehensive school health education curriculum promotes sexual abstinence as the only acceptable option for unmarried adolescents based upon the district board's belief in the importance of adolescents' acquiring necessary skills for emotional growth and maturity before making a commitment to a sexual relationship. Because most students in the district do not continue their formal education beyond high school and many young people marry soon after leaving high school, the district believes its responsibility includes providing students with information about critical topics that can assist with later life decisions and responsibilities. For this reason, family planning, including birth control and contraception, is addressed in the curriculum. Other critical topics include abortion, homosexuality, masturbation, pornography, rape, and sexual harassment. Because of the controversial nature of these topics curriculum materials are scientifically based; approved by a broad representation of community leaders, including parents, school personnel and the School Board of Polk County; and include specific guidelines for teachers to follow. Parents are encouraged to discuss the curriculum with their children and their teachers. If parents choose to exclude their children from some elements of the curriculum, the district provides an alternative learning experience in place of the excluded components of the Human Growth and Development Curriculum.

STAFF TRAINING

The district trains all teachers who teach the curriculum. Eleven nurses teach "nurse lessons" while teachers teach other health lesson blocks. To ensure that students receive a consistent message regarding health lessons, all school employees go through a "critical issues" training whether they teach the curriculum or not. Training is offered to all new staff as needed.

San Francisco Sexuality Instruction Policy

The San Francisco Unified School District includes the following guidance for sexuality instruction in its health education policy:

The instructional materials related to sexuality will be previewed by the Family Life Education Advisory Subcommittee to assure that the content is age-appropriate, culturally sensitive, language specific, inclusive of the needs of groups within the student population, and reflects the needs of the community. Membership of the Family Life Education Advisory Subcommittee will include a minimum of three parents who currently have students enrolled in the School District and are representative of the ethnicity of the student population.

As required by California Education Code (51550), if instruction addresses human sexuality, parents/guardians will be notified prior to the instruction, given the option of excluding their students from the instruction, and be given an opportunity to review the materials to be used. Also as required by California Education Code (52551), instruction about human sexuality will emphasize that the 100 percent safe way to prevent pregnancy and sexually transmitted diseases is to abstain from sexual intercourse (abstinence).

Individuals and agency representatives who make classroom presentations about human sexuality and sexually transmitted diseases will comply with California Education Codes and School District policies that include prior review by the Family Life Education Advisory Subcommittee, prior notification of parents/guardians, making instructional content and materials available for parent review, and obtaining prior approval of designated District and school site personnel. Classroom teachers who are hosting guest speakers will:

(1) preview the presentation and/or material to be used;

(2) obtain prior school site administration approval in the same manner done with all classroom visitors;

(3) when the presentation is about human sexuality, send prior notification to parents/guardians;

(4) when requested by the parent/guardian, exclude students from the instruction and provide an alternative learning activity;

(5) remain in the classroom when guest presenters are not School District employed credentialed teachers;

(6) maintain order in the classroom; and

(7) provide discipline when needed.

NEA'S Sex Education Policy

The National Education Association believes that the developing child's sexuality is continually and inevitably influenced by daily contacts, including experiences in the school environment. The Association recognizes that sensitive sex education can be a positive force in promoting physical, mental, emotional, and social health and that the public school must assume an increasingly important role in providing that instruction. Teachers and health professionals must be qualified to teach in this area and must be legally protected from censorship and lawsuits.

The Association urges that formal sex education should include parent/guardian/caregiver orientation and be planned and implemented with careful attention to developmental needs, appropriateness to community settings and values, and respect for individual differences.

The Association also believes that to facilitate the realization of human potential, it is the right of every individual to live in an environment of freely available information and knowledge about sexuality and encourages affiliates and members to support appropriately established sex education programs. Such programs should include information on sexual abstinence, birth control and family planning, diversity of culture, diversity of sexual orientation, parenting skills, prenatal care, sexually transmitted diseases, incest, sexual abuse, sexual harassment, the effects of substance abuse during pregnancy, and problems associated with and resulting from pre-teen and teenage pregnancies.

One School's Human Sexuality Program

A middle school family and consumer education teacher in Minnesota teaches a 13-period human sexuality program. Elements of each 85-minute period include:

1) inviting high school juniors and seniors in the 4H-sponsored Project 4 Teens program to role play situations involving sex and substance abuse;

2) a presentation by a health professional on how STDs are spread and treated;

3) a parenting teen and, when available, a teen who chose adoption; and

4) a discussion about healthy sexual relationships with a team from a local sexual assault clinic. Students are required to complete a project such as a scrapbook, poster, or videotape that demonstrates their understanding of issues such as sexual relationships, sexual responsibility, and goals for the future. The teacher invites students to place questions in a coffee can. She answers these questions in class or privately, depending upon their nature. When students try to embarrass people with sexual language, the teacher points out that this is a form of sexual harassment.

To gain support for the program, the teacher met with clergy, parents, and school staff. She agreed not to include information about contraception although she discusses condom use in the context of AIDS prevention. While she does not initiate discussions about abortion or homosexuality, the community does not object when these issues are addressed in response to students' questions. Before teaching the course the teacher sends a letter inviting parents to attend a meeting. Out of 300 students no more than 10 parents are likely to attend. Typical parent questions include "What is included in the program?" and "What are students responsible for completing?" According to the teacher, the most important element of gaining community support is to "put it out there and make it more open."

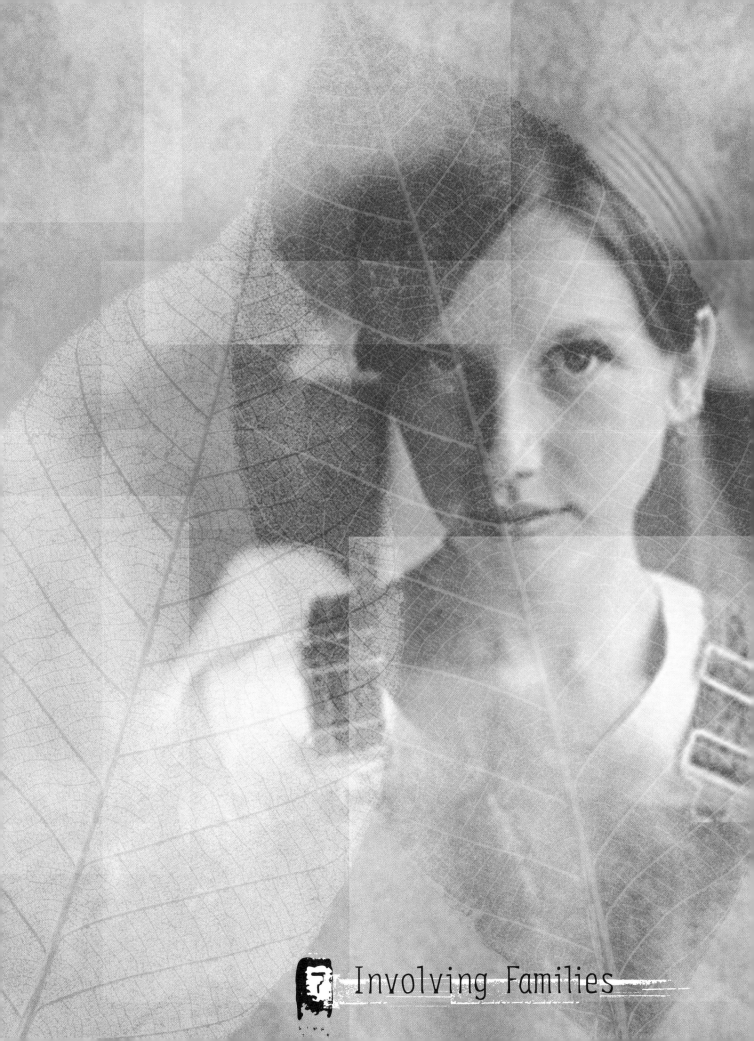

Involving Families

The Role of Parents

Children whose parents have high expectations for school success and behavior, model positive behaviors, and, most importantly, instill in their children a sense of belonging to family, school, and community are much less likely to engage in risky behaviors. Parents are students' first and foremost teachers and play the most vital role in influencing their children's lives. This is true even for teens. Contrary to popular perceptions, parents are more influential than peers and other possible influences such as TV, teachers, or siblings when it comes to making decisions about sex. In response to a poll conducted by the National Campaign to Prevent Teen Pregnancy (2004) more than two-fifths (45%) of teens ages 12-14 identified parents or guardians as most influential with peers ranking second at approximately 31% *(The National Campaign to Prevent Teen Pregnancy, 2004)*.

Keys to Successful Family Involvement

Programs that successfully involve families employ the following key activities:

* assess families' needs and interests about ways of working with the school
* have clear, measurable objectives based on family and community input
* hire and train a family liaison who is bilingual, if necessary, and sensitive to family and community needs
* inform families, businesses, and communities about family involvement policies and programs through a variety of mechanisms, including newsletters, slide shows, videotapes, speakers, and local newspapers
* recognize the importance of the community's historic, ethnic, linguistic, or cultural resources
* recruit family members as volunteers in the school
* provide staff development to teachers, administrators, and other school staff on ways to effectively partner with each other and with families
* ensure access to information about programs, services, and support available in schools and community agencies
* are flexible in scheduling activities to meet the needs of diverse families
* evaluate and adapt family involvement activities regularly

—adapted from National Coalition for Parent Involvement in Education.

"Kids are very eager to learn and want to know what is true and what is false. They want to know from someone who knows what is going on. First, you have to know the facts, and, second, be honest with them. If you don't know something, tell them you'll check. Otherwise, they lose respect— they'll find the answer on the Internet or from their sisters and brothers." (School Nurse, Mississippi)

Policymakers are becoming increasingly aware of the importance of family involvement in education. Title I, Special Education, Head Start, and other federal programs mandate collaboration with families. Many state and district policies also contain directives to involve families.

Parent/Child Communication

"We have done so little in primary prevention. Are we simply trying to reduce births to teens or are we trying to help kids lead better lives? We know that children whose parents talk to them do better. We need to educate parents to be sex educators."
(Program Director, Maryland)

The Impact of Parental Communication

Parents sometimes think that their opinions have no influence on their children, particularly when young people are constantly bombarded by sexually explicit images and content from the media. Although the influence of peers and the media upon children increases as they grow older, research shows that young people do want to have open discussions with their parents or a trusted adult. When students were asked with whom they would feel comfortable speaking about sex and relationships, about half of all teens said their parents. More than four out of five reported that what their parents might think influenced decisions about relationships and sexual activities *(National Campaign to Prevent Teen Pregnancy, 2004)*. Below are some responses teens gave when asked what they want to hear from parents and other trusted adults *(The National Campaign to Prevent Teen Pregnancy, 1999)*:

* Show us why teen pregnancy is such a bad idea.

* Talk to us honestly about love, sex, and relationships.

* Telling us not to have sex is not enough.

* Whether we're having sex or not, we need to be prepared.

* If we ask you about sex or birth control, don't assume we are already having sex.

* Pay attention to us before we get into trouble.

* Sometimes all it takes not to have sex is not to have the opportunity.

* We really care what you think, even if we don't always act like it.

* Show us what good, responsible relationships look like.

* We hate "The Talk" as much as you do.

Helping Parents Improve Communication Skills

Despite both parents' and children's desire to have these critical conversations, in many instances they are either not taking place or are occurring in limited detail and frequency. Recognizing how important open parent-child communication is to the health and behavior of young people, more and more attention is being paid to parent education programs as a key teen pregnancy prevention strategy. Parent-child communication programs help parents and their children talk about a range of important topics, including puberty and sexuality, alcohol and drug use, peer pressure, media messages, violence, and character.

Providing parents with opportunities to improve their communication skills can help ensure that students are receiving messages that are consistent with those that they are getting in school and that will help them make healthy decisions.

Parental influence can be a very strong preventive factor, as evidenced by numerous studies on parent-child communication. The quality of parent-child communications about sex and sexuality is a determinant of teen sexual behavior. One study in particular found that open, skilled discussions between parents and teens about sexuality were associated with an increased likelihood of teens' condom use and of discussions about sexual risk between teens and their partners *(Whitaker, Mieler, May, and Levin, 1999)*.

Advice on Talking About Sex with Your Kids

* Explore your own attitudes. The more you examine the subject, the more comfortable you will be discussing it.

* Start early. Beginning as early as possible, use an honest, continuous flow of information.

* Take the initiative. Look for opportunities or teachable moments to bring the subject up even if a child hasn't started asking questions yet.

* Talk about more than the "birds and the bees." Besides the biological facts, children really need to understand about the emotional aspects of a sexual relationship.

* Give accurate, age-appropriate information. What you say should fit the age and developmental stage of your child.

* Anticipate the next stage of development. To reduce children's anxiety, talk with them about their current developmental stage, and also what will happen during the next stage.

* Communicate your values. Your children may not always adopt your values, but they will want to know your values about sex as they struggle with how they should behave.

* Talk with your child of the opposite sex. Don't let gender differences make subjects like sex taboo. Consult with books or close friends or relatives who may help you feel more comfortable.

* Relax. You may not know all the answers, but what's more important is how you respond, not what you know.

—From Talking With Your Kids About Tough Issues (http://www.talkingwithkids.org)

The National Campaign to Prevent Teen Pregnancy offers the following tips for parents:

* Be clear about your own sexual values and attitudes.

* Talk with your children early and often about sex, and be specific.

* Supervise and monitor your children and adolescents.

* Know your children's friends and their families. Girls whose friends have poor relationships with their parents are at greatest risk for earlier sexual activity (Bearman & Bruckner, 1999).

* Discourage early, frequent, and steady dating.

* Take a strong stand against your daughter dating a boy significantly older than she is and don't allow your son to develop an intense relationship with a girl much younger than he is.

* Help your teenagers to have options for the future that are more attractive than early pregnancy and parenthood.

* Let your kids know that you value education highly.

* Know what your kids are watching, reading, and listening to.

* Strive for a relationship that is warm in tone, firm in discipline, and rich in communication—one that emphasizes mutual trust and respect.

Family Involvement Activities

Parents' lack of understanding for a program can quickly undermine it. Many states and districts have regulations that require parental permission. Whether required or not, parental support is key. However, getting parents to come to a meeting to learn about a program, ask questions, and have an opportunity to express concerns is not always easy. It requires effort and creativity. Try the following strategies:

* Make materials available for examination in the school media center, the classroom, family resource center, or other places that are accessible to parents.

* Offer an orientation at a back-to-school night or other time that is convenient for parents. If offered in the evenings, provide dinner and child care. If one large organization or site employs many parents of school-aged children in the community, make arrangements to go to the work site and do an orientation at lunch.

* Arrange for neighborhood gatherings or "coffee klatches." Parents appreciate the "support group" feel of opportunities to share their experiences with other parents.

* Cooperate with Family Resource Centers which attract and involve parents by providing services such as English as a second language classes, individual guidance on family problems, family recreational activities, and peer support groups.

* Use mailed and e-mailed notices, articles in the newspaper, or even personal phone calls.

* Be available to parents. Give parents an opportunity to express their concerns and obtain answers to their questions by phone, writing, e-mail, or a school web site.

Questions may emerge at any time as a result of students mentioning class activities or discussions, parents sharing impressions of what they think their children are learning, or parents having concerns about their children's behaviors or attitudes. Providing timely and appropriate responses to these concerns can help to maintain parental involvement and support for programs.

Ideas from the Field

A program in Maryland had a drawing for a VCR as an incentive to get parents to come to an informational meeting. The agenda included a video showing parents who did not set limits. Program organizers performed role plays and gave a copy of the video to every parent to take home to watch and discuss with their children.

One teacher says the best way to get parents involved is to involve their children. In addition to offering food, incentives and childcare, hold separate sessions for parents and children but at the same place and time.

A parent educator in Washington State markets parent workshops in workplaces, churches, community centers, youth sporting events, and through other parents. Parents who attend are rewarded with name recognition in a local newspaper or church bulletin, or win a "family night out" package that might include discount tickets for movies, ice cream, restaurants, miniature golf, etc.

A parent outreach program in a Virginia school district provides interpreters for non-English speaking parents and also sets up buddy systems for parents to use to call and remind one another about an upcoming workshop or even accompany each other to the session.

Offering Parents Options

Most state education policies include an opt-in or opt-out provision that allows families to release their children from any portion of health or sexuality education *(National Association of State Boards of Education, 1998)*. School districts generally suggest alternative programs for students whose parents choose not to grant permission for participation. For example, Montgomery Blair High School in Silver Spring, Maryland *(http://www.mbhs.edu)* offers students the following options:

* **Abstinence only.** Students assigned this unit receive information about sexual abstinence and no information about methods of contraception.

* **Self-esteem, personal and family relationships, and environmental health.** Students assigned this unit receive no information about human sexuality.

* **Independent study project.** Students assigned this project are required to select and complete an independent study project on a health-related topic.

Sample Letter to Parents

Dear Parent or Guardian:

Helping young people to develop healthy relationships and understand the responsibilities of adulthood is a concern for us all—families, school staff, and community members. This semester the Family Life Education class will address reproductive health, building healthy relationships, abstinence, refusal skills, pregnancy prevention, AIDS, and other sexually transmitted diseases. This program is designed to help students develop the knowledge, skills, and attitudes they need to prepare for responsible adult relationships.

Families need to be familiar with classroom materials so that they will be prepared to answer their children's questions and reinforce or supplement program content. Without the support and cooperation of families this program cannot work.

We invite you to attend a meeting at (date, place) to learn about and have an opportunity to comment on our program. The meeting will begin promptly at (time) and end no later than (time). Child care and a light supper will be provided.

If, after you attend this meeting, you choose not to allow your child to participate, the district will make arrangements in consultation with you for an alternative class. If you are unable to attend, the curriculum will be available for your review in the library. If you have questions, please feel free to contact me at ....

Sincerely,

Resources

Ten Tips for Parents to Help Their Children Avoid Teen Pregnancy and *Talking Back: Ten Things Teens Want Parents to Know About Teen Pregnancy* are available from The National Campaign to Prevent Teen Pregnancy, Phone: (202) 478-8500, Website: http://www.teenpregnancy.org.

How to Talk with Your Child About Sexuality: A Parent's Guide

The Facts of Life—A Guide for Teens and Their Families

Kids and AIDS: A Guide for Parents

Human Sexuality: What Children Should Know and When They Should Know It

All About Sex: A Family Resource on Sex and Sexuality are available from Planned Parenthood Federation of America, Inc.,

The April 2000 edition of ReCAPP *(Resource Center for Adolescent Pregnancy Prevention)* focuses on Parent-Teen Communication about Sexuality:

http://www.etr.org/recapp/column/column200004.htm

Talking with Kids about Tough Issues (booklet) by the Henry J. Kaiser Family Foundation *(www.kff.org)* and Children Now *(www.childrennow.org)*. For information call: *(510) 763-2444*

Ten Talks Parents Must Have with Their Children About Sex and Character by Pepper Schwartz Ph.D. and Dominic Cappello, 2000. See: *http://www.tentalks.com/*

Finding Our Voices: Talking with Our Kids about Sexuality and AIDS (booklet) Mothers' Voices United to End AIDS *(http://mothersvoices.org)*

Askable Parent (booklet), American Social Health Association *(http://www.ashastd.org)* *(919) 361-8400*

An interactive website *http://www.itsyoursexlife.com* offers teenagers information on pregnancy, contraception, and sexually transmitted diseases, stressing abstinence as the best way to prevent pregnancy but also featuring descriptions of birth control devices such as condoms and birth control pills. It offers advice on communicating in relationships; tips on how to talk about sex, contraception, STDs, etc.; and tips on talking to parents or partners about sex. Its goal is to help teens make smart sexual decisions.

A website for parents (*http://www.talk-ingwithkids.org*) offers parents advice on how to talk with their kids about sex, HIV/AIDS, violence, alcohol, and drug abuse. Parents can join an online forum or download or order booklets and a tool kit to plan events in their communities.

A website *(http://www.wordscanwork.com)* of resources from highly-respected author Jeanne Clarke.

Can We Talk?

is a four-part interactive workshop series that can help families with children in grades 4-9 talk about self-esteem, puberty and sexuality, mixed media messages, and peer pressure. The workshops also include information about human reproduction, teen pregnancy, and HIV/AIDS. They are appropriate for evening sessions in neighborhood schools and community centers or as brown bag lunch presentations in the workplace. The package contains all the tools needed to promote and facilitate the workshops and can be customized to fit every community's unique needs. The kit, which consists of a planning and training manual, family activity book, video, and tote bag is available for $75 plus shipping and handling. A Spanish-language adaptation, "Conversamos," is also available. For information about the kit or to plan a training in your school or community, call the National Education Association Health Information Network at (202) 822-7570 or visit http://www.canwetalk.org.

Ideas from the Field

A program in Iowa includes a questionnaire that students take home to discuss with parents or caregivers questions such as:

* How should teenagers show affection to someone they love?

* Should adolescents have sex with someone they love if they plan to marry them?

* What are the best kinds of protection for teenagers who are sexually active?

* What should parents do to help their child avoid pregnancy or HIV infection?

Students fill in how they think their parents would answer and then talk to their parents to see how close they came.

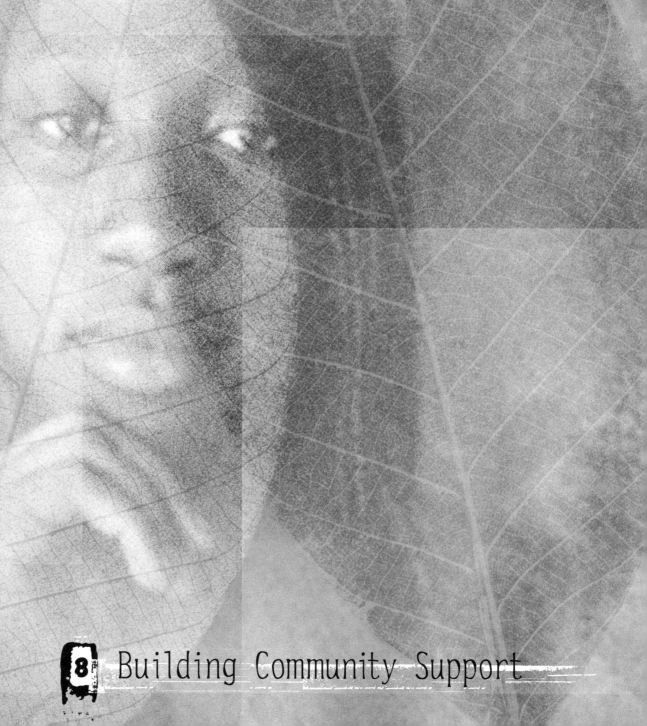

8 Building Community Support

How a Community Coalition Can Help

Most successful teen pregnancy prevention programs draw upon the combined efforts of diverse individuals in the community. Such individuals might include parents and other family members, community organizations, health and mental health providers, businesses, the faith community, the school board, school administrators, teachers, students, and other school personnel. Active participation by these individuals constitutes a "community coalition." If the community already has a school health committee, teen pregnancy prevention efforts need to be coordinated with that group's activities. Since academic achievement has such a strong relationship to teen pregnancy, involvement of the school improvement committee is highly desirable.

A community coalition that targets teen pregnancy can:

* **Broaden the base of support** for teen pregnancy prevention efforts by working with a broad range of community institutions (including public health departments, social service agencies, youth and families, business, health care, local media, faith organizations, education, philanthropy, hospitals, and universities) and engaging these new partners on an ongoing basis.

* **Ensure that students hear a consistent message by developing a message** with input from adults and teens based on a core set of values such as honesty, courage, respect, and responsibility. A theme might be to delay sexual intercourse until they are emotionally mature, economically secure, and in a long-term relationship. Examples of messages developed by other communities are: "It is important to finish high school," "It is a lot easier to finish high school if you don't have to care for a child," "Make the smart choice. Don't have sex until you are ready," and "It is appropriate to refuse unprotected sex."

* **Promote community awareness, support, and involvement** by holding public forums; cultivating relationships with the media so that coverage is educational rather than sensational or controversial; establishing a speakers' bureau that includes representatives of the PTA, teens, business, and the faith community; and offering media literacy workshops that address how media use sexuality to promote product sales and entertainment programs.

* **Reflect community concerns** by giving a cross-section of the community opportunities to voice its opinions.

* **Secure resources to carry out activities.**

Two Useful Resources for Building Community Support

A Comprehensive Approach to Reduce Pregnancy and the Spread of HIV: An Advocacy Kit includes a presentation script with overhead transparency masters and tips for coalition building. Available for $24.95 plus shipping from the American School Health Association, 7263 State Route 43, P.O. Box 708, Kent, OH 44240. Phone: (330) 678-1601 Website: http://www.ashaweb.org

Putting What Works to Work (PWWTW) is a project of the National Campaign to Prevent Teen Pregnancy funded, in part, by the Centers for Disease Control and Prevention. Through PWWTW, the Campaign translates research on teen pregnancy prevention and related issues into user-friendly materials for practitioners, policymakers, and advocates. Reports, issue briefs, and presentation materials prepared as part of PWWTW are available online at www.teenpregnancy.org/works/default.asp .

Organizing a Community Coalition

An advocate in Maryland spent the first year of pregnancy prevention program development sponsoring community events to raise community awareness. She targeted the community's school administrators, juvenile officers, and other influential members to help them understand the effect of teen pregnancy upon kids and recognize that pregnancy was often the result of unaddressed difficulties. Her theme was "Prevention is everybody's business— investing in prevention is less costly than the alternative."

Steps for creating a community coalition are:

* **Establish** a steering committee of key individuals. This can be a small core group that has the necessary expertise and links to the school and the broader community. As this group develops structure and concrete goals and objectives over time, it can expand to include more extensive membership.

* **Agree** on structure, process, and purpose. This requires answering questions such as: Who will coalition members be and what will be their roles? How will decisions be made? How often will the group meet and who will be responsible for calling, conducting, and reporting on meetings? What is the group's mission, i.e., its rationale

for existence and long- and short-term goals? Who will staff the coalition and what resources will support the staff?

* **Gather** data. Questions to ask are: How common is teen pregnancy in the community? What is known about young people's sexual behavior and the occurrence of sexually transmitted diseases? Which teens appear to be most at risk? What community programs and services currently address teen pregnancy? What does the community believe about teen pregnancy?

* **Analyze** the data. Where are the largest concentrations of teen pregnancy? What factors appear to contribute? What prevention strategies is the community likely to support? What existing resources can the coalition build upon?

* **Develop** a plan. Create goals and objectives, decide who will implement the plan, when identified tasks will be accomplished, and what resources will be required. Use Chart III: Community Action Plan in the appendix to record your plan.

* **Identify funding/resources.** Schools cannot be solely responsible for preventing teen pregnancy and meeting the needs of pregnant and parenting teens. Departments of health and community agencies often have resources for working cooperatively with schools. Suggestions for identifying potential sources appear in the "Finding Resources" section of this chapter.

* **Implement the plan.** A well-defined plan includes discrete tasks and a timeline for accomplishing each task. Be realistic about what can be accomplished. Early, small successes demonstrate to coalition members and to the community that this effort can be effective. Schedule opportunities for reporting, receiving feedback, and celebrating successes to maintain momentum.

* **Keep** the community informed. Strategies for informing schools include posters, displays and special projects, announcements over the public address system, e-mail or website communications, articles in the school newspaper or newsletter, and special events such as health fairs. Develop a positive relationship with the media; consider inviting a representative of the media to join the coalition.

* **Evaluate** progress. Annual evaluations of project goals and how well they are being addressed help keep programs on track. An evaluation component can ensure continued funding and community support, particularly if findings demonstrate that the program is 1) making a difference and 2) saving money. The groundwork for evaluation is laid at the very beginning during the data collection process when needs are identified and plans are made. Ongoing (process) evaluation can help to determine what is working and what modifications are needed. Evaluation strategies can include observations, interviews, surveys, reviewing records, and feedback at meetings.

Measuring the effects or outcomes of activities (outcome evaluation) can be more complicated. It might be difficult to demonstrate that a reduction in teen pregnancy is the result of a particular program rather than other factors in students' lives.

Evaluation specialists at local colleges or universities or state departments of education or health may be willing to assist either as part of a graduate program or for a reasonable fee.

Sample Plan

Mission Statement:

To reduce the teen pregnancy rate in our community by providing teens with greater knowledge of work and education opportunities available to them and by strengthening policies and programming.

Goals:

1. To reduce the number of teenagers who are sexually active.

2. To increase the number of sexually active teenagers who are able to access family planning.

3. To increase the number of businesses and other community groups who partner with local schools to expand student access to mentoring and work experiences as well as to college scholarships.

Objectives:

1. By January, 500 additional adolescents in need of family planning services will have access to care through a system of coordinated clinics in the community.

2. By January, 350 students will be matched to mentoring and job shadowing opportunities in the community.

From National Campaign to Prevent Teen Pregnancy (1999) Get Organized

Sample Plan 2

The following was adapted from an example developed by the American School Health Association (1997).

Goal:

To increase the number of high school students who abstain from unprotected sexual intercourse by 20%.

Objective 1:

By the end of one year, 80% of ninth-grade students will be able to describe the process of reproduction and identify several ways to prevent pregnancy and STDs.

Objective 2:

By the end of one year, 80% of ninth-grade students will be able to demonstrate effective skills to resist pressures to engage in sexual intercourse.

Objective 3:

By the end of six months, all ninth-grade health teachers will be able to use a variety of teaching methods that actively engage students in the learning process.

Objective 4:

By the end of one year, two health services facilities located at or near high schools will provide pregnancy prevention and STD diagnosis and treatment services specifically designed to meet the needs of adolescents.

Suggested strategies include:

* the district adopting policies requiring sexuality education that includes skill development and factual content.

* the district adopting and obtaining a curriculum that meets predetermined criteria such as those in Chapter 5.

* teachers attending a training on the adopted curriculum that includes practicing teaching social skills

* a community meeting that addresses ways families and school staff can reinforce lessons learned in the classroom

A Community-wide Initiative

The School Community Program for Sexual Risk Reduction Among Teens in South Carolina was initiated in 1982 on the premise that teen pregnancy reduction requires multiple interventions and community-wide participation, including schools, community agencies, media, faith leaders, health and social services professionals, parents, and youth organizations. In the second year of implementation the estimated pregnancy rate for girls ages 14-17 dropped from 66.9 to 24.0 per 1,000. Major program components include

(1) strengthening sexuality education by training teachers, community members, and agency professionals;

(2) age-appropriate, comprehensive K-12 sexuality education;

(3) linkages with health care providers to increase access to services;

(4) regular meetings with school administrative staff, parent advisory groups, health councils, and others involved in school health decisions;

(5) increased public awareness through the media;

(6) training and support for peer leaders;

(7) alternative activities for youth;

(8) programs in religious organizations; and

(9) networking with interagency councils and social agencies.

The program was initially funded by a five-year grant to the University of South Carolina School of Public Health from the Office of Adolescent Pregnancy Programs, U.S. Department of Health and Human Services, then by the South Carolina Health and Human Services Finance Commission through community block grant funds, and more recently by Medicaid Family Planning fee-for-services programs. The program has been replicated in three Kansas communities with grants from the Kansas Health Foundation. For more information about this program, including implementation steps, obtain the publication *Implementation Standards and Guidelines for Community-Based Projects: Lessons Learned from the School/Community Sexual Risk Reduction Project* by writing to: Murray Vincent, Ed.D., Department of Health Promotion and Education, School of Public Health, University of South Carolina, Columbia, South Carolina 29208. (http://www.socio.com/srch/summary/pasha/full/passpp01.htm)

Building Consensus

Programs that address sexual content can provoke discussion and controversy. Questions might emerge from individuals and organizations inside and outside the school community, particularly regarding possible conflict between these programs and the roles of parents and faith communities. Most community members will agree that preventing teen pregnancy is a desirable goal. How to achieve this goal, however, can be a source of disagreement. To gain support for a proposal, proponents need to arm themselves with

1) evidence that what is being suggested works,

2) support from others in the education and broader communities, and

3) a willingness to be flexible and hear what others have to say.

Maintaining Accord

While conflict cannot always be avoided, here are some suggestions for reducing the possibility and addressing it when it happens:

* Keep the effort focused on the shared goal of teen pregnancy prevention. Avoid getting sidetracked on issues such as abortion or premarital sex.

* Base decisions on sound research. Invite experts to provide reliable, accurate explanations.

* Plan to make a long-term commitment. This will provide the opportunity to pursue a variety of strategies in case some do not work or become embroiled in controversy.

* Organize a broad-based, inclusive coalition that will give all interested parties a voice.

* Identify respected people as leaders. Ask a skilled facilitator to conduct meetings.

* Obtain agreement on clear ground rules and policies for conducting meetings, making decisions, bringing in new people, and working with the media.

* Summarize the discussion from each meeting in writing, including points of consensus and disagreement with follow-up action steps.

* Develop shared understanding by learning together. Conduct program site visits together or invite experts to speak to the group about specific strategies or programs.

* Take early successful action. Completing something that everyone supports will motivate people and generate support for activities.

(National Campaign to Prevent Teen Pregnancy, 1999a; Marx & Northrop, 1995)

Depending upon the climate in the community, proponents might want to focus on "youth development" activities rather than "sexuality education programs" in their initial proposal. Sexuality education programs concentrate on reducing sexual risk-taking by addressing specific behaviors that might result in pregnancy, HIV infection, or other STDs. Youth development programs do not focus on young people's problems or risky behaviors but rather on developing young people's potential and helping them feel and become competent. These programs aim to strengthen self-esteem, improve skills, and provide opportunities for growth and achievement in a setting where young people can have meaningful relationships with adults and older peers. People who disagree over approaches to sexuality education can often agree on youth development as an intervention that might motivate teens to avoid pregnancy *(National Campaign to Prevent Teen Pregnancy, 1998a)*.

Involving the Faith Community

The U.S. Constitution's principle separating church and state is sometimes used as an argument for not involving the faith community in school programs. However, both sides have come to realize the enormous contribution that faith communities can make to help prevent teen pregnancy. Because the "religious right" has challenged some educational programs, many public school administrators and proponents of public education mistakenly assume that these views reflect those of the larger religious community and hesitate to seek faith involvement. Some faith leaders are realizing that they need to communicate other views and not allow the religious right to speak for the entire religious community *(Comprehensive Health Education Foundation, 1995)*.

The National Campaign to Prevent Teen Pregnancy (1999) recommends involving the faith community in preventing teen pregnancy because faith communities:

* focus on values. Adolescents involved in religious activities are more likely than other teens to delay sexual activity.

* have community credibility. Many religious organizations are already positively involved in a range of activities that affect the life of the community.

* involve young people, parents, and potential volunteers. Most faith communities offer a variety of programs for young people. Parents who are active in a congregation

are likely to be active in the lives of their children. Faith communities frequently have a tradition of community service and can be a source of skilled volunteers for key activities such as mentoring or public speaking.

* have conflict resolution skills. Many religious leaders strive to find common ground among people with diverse views and can help identify points of agreement and bridge differences related to activities targeting teen pregnancy prevention. Communities frequently have interfaith coalitions that can provide a forum for resolving controversies.

* can provide in-kind contributions. Faith communities can provide space for meetings or other activities, announcements in newsletters, volunteers, and similar support.

Faith communities can support teen pregnancy prevention both within their own congregations and through involvement in or support of a community coalition. The National Campaign to Prevent Teen Pregnancy offers nine tips for faith leaders to address teen pregnancy within their communities. School personnel can share these tips with religious leaders in their community and work with their faith communities to carry them out.

Faith Communities Can:

* Address the need teens have for spiritual fulfillment and help them find answers to the many challenging problems they face.

* Encourage parents to talk with their children about sex and morality within the context of their faith tradition.

* Enlist adults in the faith community to help young people.

* Using clear and unambiguous language, make sure children and teenagers understand what their faith tradition says about sex, love, and marriage in general and teen pregnancy, in particular.

* Learn about contemporary youth culture—what young people are reading, listening to, watching, and doing.

* Organize supervised group activities for teenagers.

* Reach out to teenagers who are not involved in a faith community.

* Celebrate achievement and excellence.

* Reach out to other faith communities, neighborhood organizations, and institutions that work with young people.

—The National Campaign to Prevent Teen Pregnancy, 1999d.

For more information about actions and resources to help faith communities work with young people around issues such as sexuality and pregnancy, see *Nine Tips to Help Faith Leaders and Their Communities Address Teen Pregnancy,* available from The National Campaign to Prevent Teen Pregnancy, 1776 Massachusetts Avenue, N.W., Suite 200, Washington, DC 20036. Website: http://www.teenpregnancy.org

Developing Legislative Support

Advocacy for teen pregnancy prevention should not stop at the school, district, or even community level. State statutes and policies often govern what can be taught and the kinds of programs that a community can offer. Legislative awareness of community needs and possibilities can influence funding for teen pregnancy prevention as well as other health-related endeavors. Some communities invite legislators or their staff to become members of their community coalition. Others provide direct contact with a program in action. Members of the Maryland School-Based Health Center Initiative invited legislators to accompany them on a visit to successful programs in a neighboring state. Subsequently, for the first time, the state legislature allocated $1.5 million to support school-based health centers. A family consumer science teacher in Washington State invited legislators to observe her class for pregnant and parenting teens and, as she put it, "they really had their eyes opened." School personnel can work with others in the state or district to organize hearings or briefings for legislators and other policymakers. Desirable sites for these events are locations with high rates of teen pregnancy or with promising programs. Involve youth, members of the faith and business community, and parents.

Tips for organizing site visits

✳ Target all policymakers from the area, including Congressmen, state legislators, mayors, city council representatives, school board members, and school administrators.

✳ Ask prominent community or business leaders to extend the invitation.

✳ Include youth in the presentation.

✳ Take pictures and distribute them widely to participants and the local press.

—The National Campaign to Prevent Teen Pregnancy, 1999a

Tips for organizing a legislative briefing:

✳ Have a well-respected legislator extend the invitation to her or his colleagues.

✳ Disseminate a briefing book or fact sheet with county and city data.

✳ Hold legislative briefings in or near the state capitol building for easy accessibility.

✳ Offer lunch or other refreshments.

✳ Invite the press.

—The National Campaign to Prevent Teen Pregnancy, 1999a

State Partnerships

A number of states have organized state-level partnerships to address teen pregnancy prevention. The Governor's Council on Adolescent Pregnancy in Maryland and the Governor's Initiative on Family and Children First in Ohio (*CCSSO, 1999*) are examples of support at the executive level. The Healthy Teen Network publishes a directory of state and local coalitions annually. Call 202-547-8814 to order a copy.

Organizations in some states have formed coalitions to promote school health. State departments of health and education and some state affiliates of the American Cancer Society and the American Alliance for Health, Physical Education, Recreation & Dance have this state-by-state information. About 20 states receive funding from the Centers for Disease Control and Prevention to develop partnerships between state departments of education and public health to develop coordinated school health programs that seek to prevent behaviors that put young people at risk. Visit the Division of Adolescent and School Health web site (*http://www.cdc.gov/HealthyYouth/index.htm*) or call state departments of education or health to find out whether a state is one of them.

Finding Resources to Support Teen Pregnancy Prevention Activities

Implementing teen pregnancy prevention activities requires materials, staff time, staff training, and other resources. To meet these needs, schools might find ways to reallocate existing funding or they might need to identify new resources. Use Chart IV: *Existing Funding for Teen Pregnancy Prevention in My Community* in appendix B to record answers to the following questions to document a school's needs:

* What resources will the program need (staff, space, materials, etc.) and what will they cost?

* What resources (monetary and in-kind) are currently in place that can be used to support these activities (e.g., health edu-

cation, Leave No Child Behind, IDEA for special needs, school health services, community programs, recreational facilities, Medicaid, volunteer programs, etc.)?

* How can they or do they complement one another?

* What are other potential sources of funding and in-kind contributions?

Funding and in-kind contributions can come from a variety of sources such as local revenues, foundations, federal or state programs, local businesses, local departments of health, health maintenance organizations, faith communities, or sympathetic members of the community. Some **district school boards** demonstrate their support for a program by including in the district budget funding for curriculum purchase or staff professional development. In some communities the **mayor's office** spearheads teen pregnancy prevention efforts and allocates funding for this purpose. In other communities **departments of public health** fund nurses who work in the schools. **Local businesses, health maintenance organizations, or other agencies** in the community that have an interest in the health and achievement of young people might provide service learning opportunities as well as financial support. Some programs obtain materials by, for example, borrowing videos from other schools, districts, or local or state health departments; or receiving donated items such as diapers or baby formula. **Fitness centers** might provide access to their

Advocacy Kit

Advocates for Youth has developed an advocacy kit for organizing at the state and local level to improve adolescent reproductive and sexual health programs and policies. The kit includes information on building coalitions, conducting needs assessments, planning public education campaigns, working with the media, educating policymakers, and responding to controversy. Available online at http://www.advocatesforyouth.org.

facilities for after-school activities to promote physical activity. A **business supply company** might contribute art supplies. **Employees of local businesses and organizations** might volunteer time. If the community has a sizable Medicaid population, explore with **the state Medicaid agency** the possibility of applying for Medicaid funding (*Kelly, Vincent, Barnes, Lacson, & Rao, no date*).

The Centers for Disease Control and Prevention (CDC) maintains the Healthy Youth Funding (HY-Fund) database, a regularly updated website that offers timely, accessible information about federal and foundation funding opportunities for developing or improving adolescent and school health-related programs including teenage pregnancy prevention. Go to *http://www.cdc.gov/HealthyYouth/funding/index.htm*.

Examples of federal funding that can support youth development and other activities that can reduce high risk behaviors are:

* The U.S. Department of Education funds 21st Century Community Learning Centers which are school-based centers that provide safe, supervised after-school, weekend, or summer activities for children, youth, and their families (*http://www.ed.gov/Programs/21stcclc/index.gov*).

* The U.S. Department of Agriculture provides support for nutritious snacks for after-school programs (*http://www.fns.usda.gov/cnd/afterschool/default.htm*).

* The federal welfare reform program passed in 1996 allows states to use Temporary Assistance for Needy Families (*TANF*) funds for extended learning programs when these programs prevent high risk behavior that can lead to unmarried pregnancies (one of TANF's purposes) by providing structured, productive activities for youth during out-of-school time (*Council of Chief State School Officers, 2000*). States are using TANF funds to promote quality child care, early childhood education, teen pregnancy prevention, stay-in-school initiatives, and other programs that aim to give children and youth the support they need for healthy development (*Golonka, Lovejoy, & Stebbins, 2000*). States have some degree of latitude in determining how they apply these resources.
Using TANF to Finance Out-of-School Time and Community School Initiatives published by The Finance Project, (*http://www.financeproject.org*) is a good source of information.

* The Office of Adolescent Pregnancy Programs (*OAPP*) in the U. S. Department of Health and Human Services (*http://www.opa.osophs.dhhs.gov.titleXX/oapp.html*) periodically funds Adolescent Family Life Demonstration Projects that support community-based organization efforts to create comprehensive and integrated approaches to the delivery of services to pregnant teens, teen parents, their partners, children, and extended family.

Tips for Proposal Writing

When writing a proposal, include:

* why the program is needed, including data on teen pregnancy in the community and the costs of teen pregnancy in educational, health, and economic terms

* specific needs to be addressed

* goals and objectives of the proposal

* a plan of operation

* what the program will cost. When asking for a substantial amount, avoid having the entire proposal rejected by listing costs of individual items or activities that the funder might choose to support if the total exceeds the funder's capacity.

* a plan for evaluation that will demonstrate to the funder that the resources are making a difference

* a listing of other sources of support that have already been identified, including how district educational and health resources are involved

* letters of support from respected members of the community

Applications and guidelines for submitting proposals to organizations, corporations, or foundations can be found on web sites or obtained by phone. When approaching a local organization, find out who the local manager or public affairs officer is. Learn as much as possible about the organization's or business's interests and priorities before making contact. Make sure that teen pregnancy prevention or youth development fits one of these priorities. Write a letter that states how you are proposing to address those interests and priorities. Follow up with a phone call to schedule an appointment.

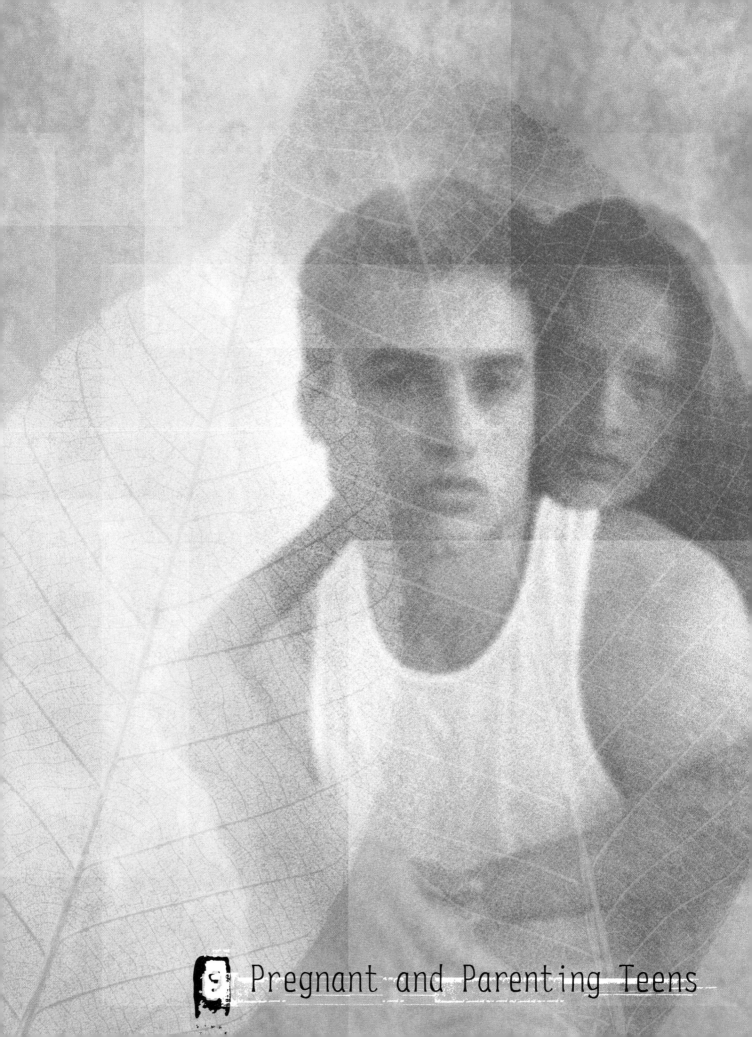

Pregnant and Parenting Teens

Pregnant and Parenting Teens

School districts need to ensure the development and implementation of policies, programs, and funding to support the health and educational outcomes of pregnant and parenting teens. Pregnant and parenting teens need multiple supports to help them develop positive parenting skills, take responsibility for their children, stay in school until graduation, and avoid another pregnancy. One third of pregnant teens receive inadequate prenatal care. One fourth of teenage mothers have a second child within two years of their first *(NELS, 1998)*. When a young person has to deal with both a toddler and an infant, going to school is unlikely to be a priority. While seven out of 10 teen mothers do complete high school, they are less likely than women who delay childbearing to go on to college *(Alan Guttmacher Institute, 1999)*. Appropriate care can result in improved support, enhanced parenting skills, encouragement to meet educational goals, and improved social outcomes for the babies and children these young parents may have in the future *(Klahn & Iverson)*.

Negative attitudes of school personnel are one of many barriers pregnant and parenting students face when striving to meet educational goals. It is not uncommon for students to be penalized for being excused from class to receive special services, arrange for child care, or other activities related to their pregnancy or parenting status. Schools need to create an environment that is free from such discrimination and ensures that no student is failed for poor attendance during childbirth and immediate postpartum *(Klahn & Iverson)*. School personnel have the power to advocate for these students and influence the policies and opinions of their colleagues so that pregnant and parenting adolescents receive the education and services they need.

Title IX of the Education Act of 1972 protects students from discrimination based on pregnancy, marital or parenting status, or gender *(U.S. Department of Education Office of Civil Rights, 1992)*. For example, under Title IX school districts cannot automatically assign pregnant or parenting students to separate schools or programs unless they have the same educational offerings and experiences available to other students *(Center of Assessment and Policy Development, 1999)*. Title IX protections need to be incorporated into school policy. A checklist created by the Center for Assessment and Policy Development *(http://www.capd.org/home/services/ teenparents/ ta_adds/weblist13.pdf)* can help school personnel determine how well their schools comply with these requirements *(Wolf, 1999)*.

From an educational perspective the needs of pregnant and parenting students can be quite similar to those of many other students who are at risk of educational failure. Consequently, committing funds to develop and implement alternative instruction methodologies and other innovative educational approaches for the benefit of teen parents can benefit a broad range of students with similar needs *(Center of Assessment and Policy Development, 1999)*.

Educational Options for Pregnant and Parenting Teens

Suggestions for improving attendance and performance

* Delayed starting times to allow time to feed and clothe their children and themselves.
* Providing space and time within the school day for social service agencies to conduct appointments.
* Limiting coursework to credits necessary for graduation.

Non-traditional strategies for meeting graduation requirements

* Awarding credits based on student's demonstration of mastery of the material rather than on the basis of attendance over the course of the school year. Students proceed at their own pace, some moving quickly while others progress toward graduation more slowly.
* Night school for students who find it difficult to attend school during traditional hours.
* Summer school and Saturday classes to make up courses or accelerate graduation.

* Home study or homebound instruction to keep students from falling behind during postpartum period or in situations where students are confined to bed for medical reasons.
* Makeup classes before or after school or during lunch period.
* Offering opportunities to enroll in courses at other institutions.
* Creative course development such as combining materials typically taught in separate classes to enable a small number of teachers to offer a wider range of classes.
* Community or school service for school credit, for example, as an aide in the library.
* Seminars, workshops, life skills training, and field trips.
* Independent study with guidance from teachers and pre- and post-tests to confirm mastery of material.
* Gaining work experience and credits by working with mentor volunteers from community organizations or business partnerships.

—Adapted from Centers for Schools and Communities, 1999.

What About the Fathers?

* An estimated 14% of high school-aged males report contributing to at least one pregnancy.

* Six percent of sexually experienced males aged 15-19 report having fathered a child (*National Campaign to Prevent Teen Pregnancy, 1999*).

* Fathers of children of teen mothers tend to be out of school or past school age. Only 26% of the men involved in pregnancies of women under age 18 are estimated to have been as young, 35% are aged 18-19, and 39% are at least 20 (*The Alan Guttmacher Institute, 1994*).

* Older men involved in a teen pregnancy are less likely to have completed high school and are more likely to be unemployed.

While some teen males and some young men have sex with significantly younger girls, they represent a small minority (*National Campaign to Prevent Teen Pregnancy, 1999*). Most sexually experienced teen males have sexual partners close to their own age—the average difference is less than six months. Most teenage girls report first male sexual partners as someone they have dated for a while who is relatively close to their own age—on average, only two to three years older. The closer in age teen partners are, the more likely they are to have used contraception at first sex. This helps to explain why those girls who have sex with older men are more likely to become pregnant. As age differences increase, condom use

The Thurston House Fatherhood Initiative in Meadville, Pennsylvania is an example of how local service providers implement ELECT (Education Leading to Employment and Career Training), a state program for pregnant and parenting teens. The agency provides teen fathers with the opportunity to get together to learn, network, support one another, and apply what they learn in their homes and community. Program goals include:

* Increase awareness of the importance of fathers in their children's lives

* Strengthen families

* Foster better relationships between fathers, children, and their families

* Encourage parental responsibility

* Establish paternity

* Prepare young men to establish or increase support for the child

* Establish or increase visitation or access to the child

* Coordinate access to services such as legal assistance, employment, and training opportunities

Address: 870 Thurston Road, Meadville, PA 16335, Phone: (814) 724-6768

declines. This may be attributed to differences in the balance of power and the communication and negotiation that occurs within the relationship (*Moore, Driscoll, & Ooms, 1997*).

The 2001 Youth Risk Behavior Survey (YRBS) conducted by the Centers for Disease Control and Prevention confirms these findings. According to the YRBS, female high school students in grade 12 (9.4%) were much more likely to report having been pregnant than grade 12 male high school students (4.8%) were to report that they had gotten someone pregnant. What is not known is how many young men that age had already dropped out of school and consequently were not counted, whether males knew they were responsible for someone's pregnancy, and whether males were responsible for more than one pregnancy (*Grunbaum et al., 2002*).

Rates of teen fatherhood are higher among inner-city and African American youth and among boys who engage in a combination of problem behaviors such as disruptive school behavior, drug exposure or use, and gang membership. Becoming a father does not necessarily encourage young males to become more responsible. In fact, one study found that becoming a father seemed to increase teens' delinquent behavior (*Thornberry et al., 2000*).

Case Management

School policies sometimes identify the school nurse as the case manager or team leader for activities serving pregnant and parenting teens. School nurses' medical and psychosocial training prepare them to coordinate necessary services or programs. The school nurse and/or other professional staff such as a school social worker can be involved throughout the adolescent's pregnancy and early parenting, starting with the presenting symptoms of pregnancy. At the time of diagnosis, the nurse and social worker can take a personal and social history to assess the adolescent's feelings about the pregnancy; social support systems such as family, the father, friends, teachers, counselors; history of abuse; and tobacco, alcohol, and other drug use.

If a pregnant student expresses to a school professional that she is undecided about what she wants to do, or has chosen to either terminate the pregnancy or arrange adoption, in most cases the professional will want to encourage the student to involve her parents or guardians in the decision. At this point, the school professional should rely on his/her district's policies to clarify his/her role in the matter. See also Chapter 4, "Confidentiality."

Policy Statement

An agreement between the Multnomah County, Oregon, health department and the school district is an example of a policy for counseling pregnant teens, including confidentiality and providing information regarding options (see page 91). The agreement recognizes that early diagnosis, referral and case management of pregnant teens leads to optimum outcomes. It prohibits on-site abortion counseling and referral by school-based health centers but does not prohibit informing pregnant teens regarding options available to them and following them until they have successfully transferred to another source of health care.

Pregnancy Counseling Policy

1. When initially counseling a client with a positive pregnancy test, the nurse, nurse practitioner, or physician's assistant is expected to assess the adolescent for:

   a. Feelings about the pregnancy

   b. Risk for suicide

   c. Knowledge of legal options available

   d. Support systems

   e. Ability to make an independent decision, which may be evidenced by behavior such as:

      1. Ability to articulate a plan

      2. Identification of a support system

      3. Ability to keep medical appointments

      4. Ability to follow medical plans

   f. Immediate physical concerns

2. If the adolescent appears to function at a mature, intellectual level, parental involvement should be encouraged and facilitated but the adolescent's right to confidentiality should be respected. The chart should document the client's wishes and the provider's criteria for deciding to breach confidentiality or not. In the case of an adolescent at high risk due to low intellectual function, emotional disturbance or poor judgment, the provider must seriously consider involving a parent or guardian. Where students are ambivalent about parent/ guardian involvement the provider should offer to mediate to enable the client to involve the parent or guardian in their care.

3. All clients should be given the opportunity for in-depth options counseling through a referral.

4. If the client's decision appears to be termination, the provider must discontinue counseling at this point and refer the student outside the SBHC.

5. In the event of a decision to continue the pregnancy, the nurse assists the client in obtaining prenatal care, insurance if necessary, and then tracks the client for follow-up and outcome data.

6. Each pregnant client should have an identified prenatal care provider outside of the SBHC. The role of the SBHC is to assess that the client is obtaining prenatal care, not to duplicate services.

7. Clients should be followed to confirm that they access the referral resource successfully. If not, the provider should consider involving a parent at this point, and coordinating tracking with the field nurse.

8. If the first prenatal appointment is delayed, the SBHC provider may decide to do an initial assessment consisting of pap, STD testing, dating parameters, Rh determination, CCMS, MSAFP or other tests appropriate to the gestation.

9. Initiate pregnancy audit tool and keep, either until the outcome of the pregnancy is known or at the latest, summer break.

Visit http://www.advocatesforyouth.org/publications/iag/cntrcptv.htm to read more about this policy.

Developing a Plan

For a student who chooses to carry a pregnancy to term, professional staff can work with the student to develop a care plan that targets both the student's health care and successful completion of the student's educational program. This might include notifying family and the father, if this has not already been done; identifying school policies regarding pregnant student absenteeism and participation in physical education, sports, and other school activities; connecting with a health care provider; providing education about pregnancy, fetal development, and preparation for delivery; and planning for the future, e.g., meeting graduation requirements, or obtaining child care.

Lack of appropriate child care can be an enormous barrier to a teen mother's continuing education. Child care can be provided in a variety of venues. It may be administered by the local school district or another community agency. A center may be located on the school site or in a nearby community facility, or the children may be cared for through a network of family child care homes. Some programs follow the school calendar while others are all day and yearlong. Schools can provide teen parents with consumer education to help them choose quality child care programs. A number of states apply resources available through the Child Care and Development Block Grant (CCDBG) to support child care programs for teen parents. Examples of programs supported by these funds can be found at *http://nccic.org/poptopics/reauthtanf.html*.

Post-partum, the staff can follow the student until graduation, providing support to prevent another pregnancy, documenting such items as class attendance and academic progress, health care provider visits, coordination of agency and other support systems, child support, and the status of the parent-child relationship, including involvement of the father (*Klahn & Iverson, no date*).

Teen parents who receive benefits under the Temporary Assistance to Needy Families (TANF) block grant are required to be enrolled in school. This is an incentive for parenting teens to stay in school or re-enroll if they have dropped out. The school social worker can ensure that students are complying with and benefiting from relevant policies and laws such as this. (See page 83 for more information about TANF.)

The State Children's Health Insurance Program (SCHIP) provides free health insurance to uninsured children whose family income meets certain eligibility guidelines. While eligibility and services covered vary from state to state, the program generally covers items such as doctor appointments, hospital stays, dental and vision services, prescription drugs, mental health care and other medical services. A baby living with his or her teen parents may be eligible for medical assistance regardless of the grandparents' income. For state-by-state information about eligibility and access to the Children's Health Insurance Program visit *http://www.cms.hhs.gov/schip/*.

Core Elements of a Comprehensive Service Strategy

Services for Adolescent Parents

* Flexible quality schooling, either in alternative settings or within comprehensive high schools, that complies with Title IX and incorporates accountability on the part of education providers

* Subsidized, accessible, reliable, quality child care while in school and during transitions between school and continued education, job training, or employment

* Pre-natal care and family planning services

* Health and nutrition counseling and services

* Case management services, including referrals to other services as needed (e.g., housing), help with transitions back to home and school, and visitation as necessary

* Family support and development services, including personal and relationship counseling for mothers and fathers

* Parenting and child development education

* Other support services, including transportation assistance, that will allow the adolescent to stay in school

* Services that facilitate transition to post-secondary education, training, or employment Visit www.nursing.umn.edu for more information.

Services for Children of Adolescent Parents

* Quality child development programming, on-site or, if off-site, in family child care homes near schools or with relatives linked to schools in such a way that children receive the same services as those in school-based care

* Preventive health care, developmental screens, and follow-up services

—Adapted from Klahn & Iverson

One of Minneapolis Public Schools' health goals is to

"Promote academic success, lifelong learning, and optimal health for pregnant and parenting adolescents and their children." The Patrick Henry High School Teenage Pregnant and Parenting Students (TAPPS) program has a support team that meets at least monthly with the school and clinic nurses, school and clinic social workers, a representative from Neighborhood TAPPS (a child care network specifically licensed to take care of these students' children), the Transition Program (an outreach program to bring dropouts back), the county adolescent parent unit, and a community outreach worker to coordinate care for these youth. Programs are reviewed and students are referred when appropriate.

The Graduation, Reality, and Dual Role Skills (GRADS) program in Vancouver, Washington evolved from a support program for pregnant and parenting students started by a high school family consumer science teacher. The principal recognized the need for such a program when an "A" student came to the teacher in tears because she was pregnant and did not know where to turn. The school nurse and a teacher from another school joined with the consumer science teacher to submit a funding proposal, which yielded $10,000 to support a school nurse. The program has now been incorporated into the school. Students participate in a daily 80-minute class that focuses on parenting skills and child abuse prevention, attend a vocational center to learn job skills, and are linked with appropriate community resources. A weekly $10 co-payment entitles enrolled students to a publicly funded child care program. The community donates toys, formula, diapers, and clothing as well as mentoring. GRADS students can waive participation in a required Current World Problems class because their program addresses similar behavioral components such as interpersonal relationships.

The Goals of the Pennsbury, Pennsylvania School District's pregnant and parenting teen program are to:

* establish collaborative relationships with community, medical, and social services to strengthen the network of support available to young parents
* help young parents develop a sense of responsibility for their future and that of their children
* encourage young parents to continue their education with graduation as an ultimate goal
* provide academic and career counseling to young parents

Grants from the March of Dimes and a local foundation pay for an instructor and some supplies. A community organization donates baby furniture, clothing, and formula for those who need them. Students meet once a week for 45 minutes during an open class period with the instructor who is based in a community organization that specializes in programs for pregnant and parenting students. Family and consumer science department teachers supplement these lessons. Twenty-five students participated in the program in 2000, three of them fathers.

The curriculum includes classes in pregnancy and childbirth, child growth and development, child care options, discipline, communication skills, community resources, career choices, job hunting, first aid, and safety. Guest speakers throughout the year address topics such as the child birthing process, breast-feeding, preventing premature birth, legal issues, career choices, and welfare issues.

—Program Coordinator

A Sample Policy for Continued Educational Support for Pregnant Students

The local school system has the responsibility to provide appropriate school programs for all students including pregnant girls, married or unmarried. These programs shall include provisions for counseling, pupil personnel work, social work, and psychological services as needed.

A girl 16 years old or older, who is pregnant, either married or unmarried, who has not completed her high school education may elect to remain in the regular school program and may not be involuntarily excluded from any part of this program. The decision to modify this program or provide an appropriate alternative educational program shall be reached in joint consultation with the girl and appropriate educational and medical personnel.

A girl who is pregnant, either married or unmarried, who is under compulsory school age, may voluntarily withdraw from the regular school program provided that she enrolls in an appropriate educational program planned for her. The decision concerning an appropriate educational program shall be reached in consultation with the girl, her parents, guardians, or husband, and appropriate educational and medical personnel.

Appropriate educational programs may be:

1. Continuation of the regular school program (modified in terms of individual needs)

2. Enrollment in a special school or special class for pregnant girls

3. Enrollment in a residential school

4. Telephone teaching

5. TV teaching

6. Home teaching

7. Programmed instruction

8. Admittance to a private maternity home

9. Combination of the above programs

It is the responsibility of the local school system working with the home to cooperate with other state, county, and city agencies, such as health, welfare, and juvenile services and with private physicians or agencies to assure that the pregnant girl receives proper medical, psychological, and social services before termination of pregnancy and for as long as needed after that.

—Adapted from Montgomery County (Maryland) Public Schools

Resources

A Resource Guide of Best Practices for Pregnant and Parenting Teen Programs is produced by the Center for Schools and Communities, a statewide initiative funded by the Pennsylvania Departments of Education and Public Welfare. This comprehensive guide describes approaches to (1) alternative educational programming, (2) school attendance and retention, (3) child care, (4) case management and family support services, (5) school-to-work programs, (6) teen father services, (7) pregnancy prevention, and (8) violence prevention. Available at *http://www.center-school.org/education/ppt/pptbest.htm* or *(717) 763-1661*.

Publications by Jeanne Warren Lindsay address many issues relevant to pregnant and parenting teens. Titles include *Surviving Teen Pregnancy, Teen Moms: The Pain and the Promise, Nurturing Your Newborn,* and *Teenage Couples: Expectations and Reality.* These and other books are available from *Morning Glory Press, 6595 San Haroldo Way, Buena Park, CA 90620 Phone: (888) 612-8254. http://www.morningglorypress.com/*

Resources for Teen Fathers

About being a father. Contact: *Channing L. Bete Company, 200 State Road, 01373-0200. Telephone: (800) 477-4776/ http://www.channing-bete.com/* $1.25 plus shipping and handling; quantity discounts available. # 49494A-5-93. Cartoon-like multicultural illustrations mainly of fathers and children (ages infant to 10) describe the responsibilities and rewards involved in being a father. Includes reasons to learn about being a father, why some fathers do not take an active role, how to understand a child's emotional needs, the ABCs of discipline, nurturing a child's mind, looking after physical health, sharing responsibilities between parents, and how to stay involved when living apart from the children. This material tested at a 7th grade reading level.

Teen dads: Rights, responsibilities and joys. Contact: *Morning Glory Press, 6595 San Haroldo Way, Buena Park, CA 90620-3748. Telephone: 888-612-8254.* Provides adolescent fathers with a guide to parenting from conception to age three, based on interviews with 41 adolescent fathers, some from the inner city and some from rural areas, some high-achievers who both work and continue their education, and others who, at the time of the interview, were in jail. Topics include providing support to one's partner during pregnancy, labor, and delivery; caring for a newborn; relationship building; and parenting.

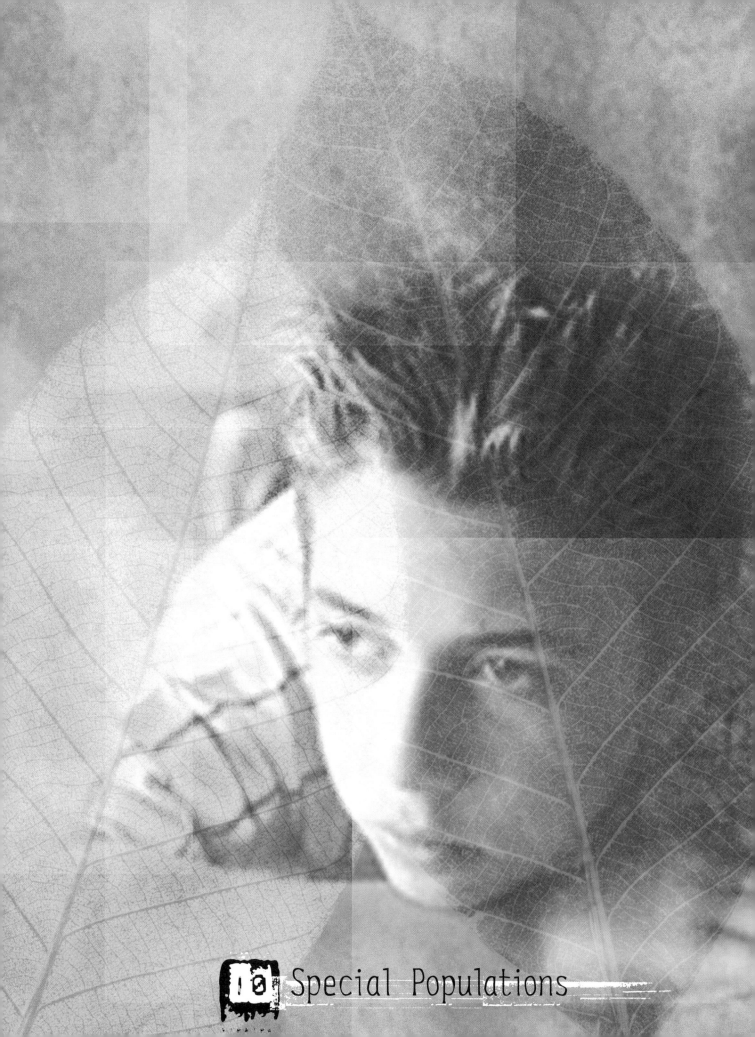

10 Special Populations

Students with Special Education Needs

"Persons with physical, cognitive, or emotional disabilities have a right to sexuality education, sexual health care, and opportunities for socializing and for sexual expression. Family, health care workers and other caregivers should receive training in understanding and supporting sexual development and behavior, comprehensive sexuality education, and related health care for individuals with disabilities." (SIECUS, 2001)

Students with special educational needs come with a wide range of conditions, including intellectual impairment (mild to severe or profound), vision or hearing impairment, learning disabilities, orthopedic (mobility) impairments, emotional disturbances, autism, and other developmental disabilities (Muccigrosso, 1994). Students with special needs are particularly vulnerable for teen pregnancy, HIV, other STDs, and sexual abuse for a number of reasons. For one, they generally know less about their bodies and their sexuality than other students because:

* Schools frequently do not include them in sexuality education classes.

* Students may not know when or whom to ask for help nor have the skills to do so.

* Few publications are written at many of these students' reading levels or accessible to students with sight or hearing deficits.

* Parents may not have communicated appropriately about these sensitive issues.

Other factors contributing to these students' vulnerability are that they

* are more likely to be misinformed because they have difficulty knowing the difference between what is real and not real.

* have little or no opportunity to learn or practice social skills.

* may have low self-esteem. Students with low self-esteem are more likely to engage in attention-getting or risky behaviors.

* may not be able to understand the consequences of what they do because they do not have well-developed decision-making skills or impulse control (*Virginia Department of Education, 1991*).

A continuum of options needs to be available for family life education instruction for students in special education. In accordance with the Individuals with Disabilities Education Act (IDEA) (P.L. 108-446) schools are required to provide students with disabilities with a "free appropriate public education" and/or related services, as needed to meet their unique learning needs. Each student with a disability who receives special education must have an Individualized Education Program (IEP). The IEP is created for that particular student and details the educational goals and objectives the student will address throughout the year. These objectives can include sexuality education.

A student's IEP is developed by school personnel, the student's parents, and (when appropriate) the student, and must be reviewed annually. The IEP team is responsible for making decisions regarding placement. Some students can receive most of their instruction in a mainstreamed class while others need instructional support from a

Tips for Teaching Students with Special Needs About Sexuality

* Establish ground rules to ensure that students feel safe to speak.

* To correct myths and misinformation, encourage students to communicate what they already know or think they know.

* Translate critical pieces of information into examples that are relevant to students' lives.

* Use cooperative learning groups, pairing more limited readers/learners with more skilled readers.

* Use frequent repetition and check in by asking students to repeat what they think they heard.

* Provide opportunities to role play situations where students have to make choices and communicate their decisions to others.

* Provide instruction and practice in assertiveness techniques such as negotiation skills and resisting peer pressure.

* Inform students where they can go for more information and help (NSBA, 1990).

 Muccigrosso, 1994

special education resource teacher. For most students with disabilities in the mild to moderate range of severity, the goals and objectives will be similar to those of regular education students at the same grade level. Others will receive instruction from an assigned special education teacher who has received special training to teach family life education. Teachers need to be familiar with the support system available in each school, including school nurses, school social workers, school counselors, and school psychologists.

Identifying Materials and Curricula for Students with Special Needs

Materials designed for regular sexuality education classes may be appropriate for some special needs students. However, special education teachers will also need to utilize a more direct teaching approach and to identify materials designed specifically for students with disabilities. Special materials may include a controlled vocabulary, high-interest low-vocabulary reading materials, captioned videos, tactual models, and more visuals, including illustrations of people with disabilities with whom students can identify (*Muccigrosso, 1994; Virginia Department of Education, 1991*).

In designing, adapting, or selecting a curriculum consider whether it:

* provides simplified but age-appropriate reading materials or media that do not require reading, hearing, vision, or mobility, depending on the student's level of ability.

* uses a variety of concrete teaching strategies to reinforce what is presented, (e.g., written materials, audiovisual materials, role play, interactive games).

* offers learning strategies that closely resemble real life situations.

* provides opportunities to interact with non-disabled peers and role models.

* reinforces learning with frequent repetition.

* takes advantage of teachable moments.

(*Adapted from Double Jeopardy: Pregnant and Parenting Youth in Special Education, ERIC/CEC Minilibrary*), http://ericec.org/

Involving Parents of Special Education Students

Parents of special education students may be more receptive to involvement in their child's sexuality education than those of nonspecial education students because they are generally more likely to be involved in their child's overall education, as part of the IEP process as well as ongoing advocacy to ensure that their child's special needs are being met. Many of these parents recognize the need to protect their child from sexual exploitation or they may be self-conscious about their child's inappropriate social behaviors. Other parents may need reassurance that sexuality education is not designed to give their child "sexual ideas" (*Muccigrosso, 1994*). As with any educational program parents should have the opportunity for ongoing review of curricula and materials. This not only gives families a chance to become familiar

with the program and provide input regarding its appropriateness for their child, but also lays the groundwork for reinforcing at home sexuality concepts learned in school. Schools can further support parents by maintaining a resource center stocked with sexuality education materials that parents can borrow.

Gay, Lesbian, Bisexual, Transgender, and Questioning Youth

According to estimates, one in 10 teenagers struggles with issues regarding sexual orientation (*Garofalo, 1998*). Sexual orientation refers to a combination of personal factors, including sexual attraction, behavior, fantasies, and emotional and social preferences (*Resource Center for Adolescent Pregnancy Prevention, 2000*). Gay, lesbian, bisexual, transgender, and questioning (GLBTQ) youth face tremendous challenges growing up physically and mentally healthy in a culture that is often unaccepting. They face emotional isolation, social rejection, and lowered self-esteem and are more likely to experience verbal abuse and physical and sexual assault than heterosexual youth, especially during their adolescence (*Ryan & Futterman, 1998*). GLBTQ youth, regardless of gender, report a prevalence of sexual abuse almost twice that of their counterparts in the general population (*Saewyc et al., 1998*). Moreover, gay and lesbian youth are four times as likely as heterosexual youth to attempt suicide (*Garofalo & Wolf, 1998*) and account for up to 30% of all completed suicides (*Gibson, 1989*).

Contrary to common perception, GLBTQ youth are at risk for teen pregnancy. Young people may feel pressured to become heterosexually active to prove to themselves and others that they are "normal" *(The Gay, Lesbian, and Bisexual Speakers Bureau, no date)*. Most GLBTQ youth actually report more heterosexual than homosexual sexual experiences. In one recent study, lesbian and bisexual girls reported more frequent heterosexual intercourse, were less likely to use effective methods of contraception, and were more likely to report involvement in prostitution than their heterosexual contemporaries. Gay and bisexual males were more likely than other males to experience early initiation of heterosexual intercourse, more frequent intercourse, and running away. The same study found a slightly higher level of pregnancy among lesbian and bisexual girls than among heterosexual girls *(Saewyc et al., 1998)*.

Females tend to identify themselves as lesbian later than males who identify themselves as gay. However, recent data suggest that female adolescents who identify themselves as lesbian are at increased risk for HIV because they are likely to engage in sexual acts with gay and bisexual males *(Rotheram-Borus, Marelich, & Srinivasan, 1999)*. GLBTQ youth have few role models to help them overcome their fear of disclosing their sexual orientation. They must decide whether their sexual partners will be of the same or opposite gender, and decide when, how, to whom, and under what circumstances to disclose their status. Consequently, GLBTQ

adolescents often seek partners outside of their local schools and neighborhoods. Leaving their neighborhoods puts them at higher risk for HIV, STDs, and pregnancy because potential partners are often found in neighborhoods or settings where a higher proportion of the population practices high-risk behaviors such as engaging in unsafe sexual practices or substance abuse. Bisexual youth may be in denial about their risk for HIV because they do not identify themselves as gay or lesbian and therefore disregard prevention messages aimed at gay youth. Lesbians might not consider themselves to be at risk because of the relatively low rate of HIV infection among lesbians as compared to gay men *(Rotheram-Borus, Marelich, & Srinivasan, 1999)*.

The entire school community—fellow students, school personnel, administration, and families— need to provide an accepting, non-discriminatory environment for GLBTQ youth and support students who might be at risk of potentially self-destructive behaviors because of their sexual orientation. Studies have shown that among GLBTQ youth, a gay or lesbian friend is often the most important person in their lives. Therefore, peer-based support and education efforts are strategies to assist GLBTQ youth. These include offering a chance to learn and practice social skills, exchange information, establish friendships and positive role models, and participate in peer support groups that address isolation, rejection, and social barriers to the healthy development of GLBTQ youth *(Garofalo, 1998)*.

Working with GLBTQ Youth

Recognize that GLBTQ youth are likely to be a part of any class or group, whether or not they are open about their identities to themselves or others. Guidelines from which all youth will benefit are:

* Always assume that 4-10% of a class is gay or lesbian (1 to 3 people in every class of 30) and that another 7-17% have an immediate family member who is gay or lesbian (another 2 to 5 people).

* Start units on sexuality defining it broadly, to include such aspects as self-esteem, gender, gender identity, gender role, gender orientation, reproductive system, sexual response system, and human needs for intimacy and belonging.

* Include in ground rules the notions of protecting others' feelings and of recognizing that there is healthy, enriching diversity within the group (specifically that no one should make assumptions about other people's family situations, sexual behavior, sexual orientation, beliefs, etc.).

* Use correct terminology when referring to people attracted to others of the same gender, i.e. "lesbian or gay woman" for a female attracted to females and "gay" for a male attracted to males. "Homosexual" is an adjective that describes sexual behavior, not people.

* Challenge abusive or derogatory terms such as "faggot."

* Use inclusive language such as "partner" instead of "boyfriend" or "girlfriend."

* Use orientation-neutral language (e.g., in 6th grade: "People get crushes at puberty." vs. "People get crushes on the opposite sex at puberty.") and inclusive language such as "Draw whomever you think of as family. That may be Mom, Dad, brothers, and sisters; it may include step-family members, foster family members, grandparents, more than one Mom or Dad, etc. Whomever you consider your family."

* Have gay/lesbian literature available in the school library and distribute a reading list. Youth may not feel ready to discuss their sexuality but may find access to literature that can help them begin to understand their sexual identity helpful.

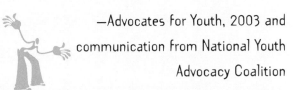

—Advocates for Youth, 2003 and communication from National Youth Advocacy Coalition

Actions Schools Can Take

⁎ Develop and publish clear policies and procedures regarding hiring practices and consequences of any acts of homophobic harassment.

⁎ Identify, develop, and advertise appropriate support services for GLBTQ youth.

⁎ Ensure that counselors and social workers have appropriate training on how to deal with the unique needs of students struggling with issues of sexual orientation and identity.

⁎ Refer students whose needs cannot be met within the school setting to appropriate community resources

⁎ Develop and support student support groups, such as gay/straight alliances.

⁎ Make readily accessible to students and their families information about resources within the school and the larger community.

—Blumenfeld, 1994

Interventions for Young Men

Just because men do not get pregnant does not mean that programs do not need to focus on them. In fact, more and more professionals are recognizing this and developing teen pregnancy prevention efforts specifically targeting young men. Adolescent men are especially at risk for unintended pregnancy and STDs because they are more likely to be misinformed about sexuality and sexual health. Young men are socialized to "know it all" when it comes to sex, to not ask questions, and to always be ready and willing to engage in sexual activity. Young men initiate sex earlier than young women and tend to have more partners over their lifetime. When combined with adolescents' sense of invulnerability, these factors result in many young men engaging in sexual activities that jeopardize the health of their partners and themselves (*Becker, 1999*).

Effective pregnancy prevention programs for young men must recognize that males at different stages of development respond to different approaches. Boys and men are more likely to make appropriate decisions about sex if they have reasons to do so. The approach needs to be age-appropriate and respectful of participants' cultural, racial, and religious backgrounds. Since males become sexually active at young ages—34% of black, 19% of Hispanic, and 14% of white male students report initiating intercourse by age 15 (*National Campaign to Prevent Teen Pregnancy, 2004*)—programs for young men need to start early. Waiting until they reach mid-adolescence is usually too late. By the time they are 15 years old they tend to reject the idea of postponing sexual involvement and begin to believe they "know everything" about contraception (*National Campaign to Prevent Teen Pregnancy, 1999a*).

Most school-based teen pregnancy prevention programs are offered to classes of boys and girls. Some sexuality education activities may be more effective when offered in groups separated by gender. Boys and young men respond to different messages and approaches than do girls and young women. To reach young men, programs need to be designed for a male audience. Moreover, male-only activities create an atmosphere of trust for participants (*Becker, 1999*). Girls may benefit from opportunities to participate in separate groups as well. Studies show that girls tend to talk less if boys are present and that even teachers with the best of intentions pay more attention to boys and give them more praise than girls (*Advocates for Youth, 1994*).

While older adults may successfully lead programs, experience suggests that the most

effective people to deliver messages to teen men are young men who are five to seven years older. The messages need to

* be concrete

* take a positive approach as opposed to scare tactics

* affirm the value of men

* avoid judgmental language about males

* differentiate between maleness and manhood

* teach young men to understand, communicate, and respect women

* help teen males overcome concerns about condom use such as embarrassment about purchasing them or discussing them with partners or that condoms will reduce physical pleasure

* connect sexual activities with having babies

(*Moore, Driscoll, & Ooms, 1997; National Campaign to Prevent Teen Pregnancy, 1999a*)

The most promising male involvement programs engage community partnerships that include local leaders, parents, service agencies, schools, faith communities, youth development programs and other community institutions. Activities described in Chapter 3 such as after-school programs, participation in sports, opportunities for community service, and mentoring relationships illustrate ways that school personnel can participate in these partnerships.

Resources

Special Education

The October 2001 edition of ReCAPP, a website maintained by ETR Associates (*http://www.etr.org/recapp*), addresses "Educating Youth with Developmental Disabilities." It features definitions of developmental disabilities, clarifies issues related to providing sexuality education to developmentally disabled young people, provides strategies for educators, and lists national organizations, websites, and resources that can provide additional information.

GLBTQ Youth

Just the Facts About Sexual Orientation & Youth, a primer for educators developed by several national organizations including NEA, is designed to help guide school personnel dealing with issues related to homosexuality in their schools, including sexual orientation development, reparative therapy, transformational ministries, and relevant legal principles. *The 2003 National School Climate Survey* sheds light on the experiences of LGBT students in America's schools. Both can be viewed on line at *http://www.glsen.org/*

From Our House to the Schoolhouse offered by Parents, Families, and Friends of Lesbians and Gays (PFLAG) is available together with other resources at *http://www. pflag.org.*

The June 2000 edition of ReCAPP, a website maintained by ETR Associates, addresses teen pregnancy prevention in relation to GLBTQ youth, featuring concise definitions of GLBTQ, an overview of relevant issues, strategies for educators, and additional resources. Click on "Archives" at *http://www.etr.org/recapp.*

The Healthy Lesbian, Gay and Bisexual Students Project of the American Psychological Association maintains a website at *http://www.apa.org/ed/lgbproj.html.*

Other websites that address issues related to GLBTQ students include:

Gay, Lesbian and Straight Education Network (*http://www/glsen.org*)

Advocates for Youth (*http://www.advocates for youth.org*)

National Youth Advocacy Coalition (*http://www.nyacyouth.org*)

Sexual Information and Education Council of the United States (SIECUS) (*http://www.siecus.org*)

Interventions for Young Men

Involving Males in Preventing Teen Pregnancy: A Guide for Program Planners discusses the importance of paternal involvement and highlights a number of fatherhood programs. Available online from the Urban Institute at *http://www.urban.org*

Male Involvement & Adolescent Pregnancy Prevention, by Robert Becker *http://www.etr.org/recapp/theories/mip/miapp/pdf*

Curricula for Special Education Students

A sampling of classroom resources for students with developmental and learning disabilities:

Middle School Through Adult

Circles I: Intimacy & Relationships—Social Distance and Relationship Building

Circles II: Stop Abuse—Helping Students Avoid Exploitation

Circles III: Safer Ways—AIDS and Communicable Disease Prevention

Life Horizons I: The Physiological and Emotional Aspects of Being Male & Female

Life Horizons II: The Moral, Social and Legal Aspects of Sexuality

Sexuality Education for Persons With Severe Developmental Disabilities

Available from: James Stanfield Co, Inc.,
Phone: (800) 421-6534
Website: http://www.stanfield.com

Curriculum for Young Men

Wise Guys
Family Life Council of Greater Greensboro
301 E. Washington Street, Suite 204
Greensboro, NC 27401
Phone: (336) 333-6890

The Virginia Department of Education has published *Family Life Education: Effective Instruction for Students in Special Education.* This 2005 publication addresses the needs of severely and profoundly cognitively handicapped, trainable mentally retarded, and mildly handicapped (e.g., educable mentally retarded, learning disabled, emotionally disturbed, visually impaired, hearing impaired, and orthopedically impaired) students. Also included is a list of publishers and resource materials for working with these populations. For information, contact the
Division of Special Education Programs, Department of Education,
P.O. Box 6Q, Richmond, VA 23216-2060
Phone: (804) 225-2880.

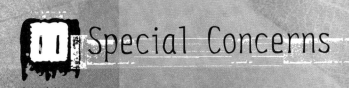 Special Concerns

Cultural Competence

Students bring to school a variety of cultural values, beliefs, and needs that can interfere with effective delivery of sexuality education. The nation's increasingly diverse student body is challenging schools to meet the needs of an increasingly pluralistic population. This situation is further complicated by the heterogeneous beliefs and value systems of students representing the dominant white, European culture. Views may differ about what constitutes a family, the roles and relationships of family members, and appropriate sexual behavior. Language used to describe matters related to sexuality such as body parts or sexual activities may differ, not only among non-English-speaking populations but also across English-speaking populations (Advocates for Youth, 1994).

School staff need to be aware of these differences and to consider, at a minimum, consulting with or involving parents or others in the community who can help to deliver appropriate messages consistent with the values and beliefs of students' families. Gaining cultural competence involves developing a mixture of beliefs, attitudes, knowledge, and skills so that one can establish trust and communicate with others, regardless of their beliefs or value systems. Becoming culturally competent requires awareness of one's own culture, values, and biases and how these affect one's view of others; being comfortable with differences between one's own culture and those of others; and recognizing when one might need assistance from someone of another culture to deal with sensitive issues. It also requires learning about the cultures of students and how these might affect their attitudes regarding sexual behaviors. Important cultural components include language and communication style, family relationships, sexuality, gender roles, religion, and economic circumstances (Advocates for Youth, 1994).

There are more than two dozen Latino cultures in the United States. Asian Americans represent over 30 different cultural groups. Black Americans include descendants of Africans brought to this continent as slaves as well as immigrants from Caribbean and African countries. Close to 300 tribes make up the Native American population. Add to this the wide variety of European ethnic groups and it is clear that no one can develop an understanding of every culture. School personnel can, however, seek to learn more about the cultures represented in their building, remaining mindful of individual differences and understanding that no one individual's view can reflect the diversity of other individuals' experiences (Advocates for Youth, 1994).

For some cultures childbearing can have a significance that conflicts with the intent of pregnancy prevention. While birthrates for white teenagers are higher in the United States than those in other Western countries, the birthrates for young African American and Latina women are even higher. For some African Americans and Latinos/Latinas who live in poverty, having children is often the only way they feel they can prove that they are socially productive and demonstrate their manhood or womanhood. Since use of condoms reduces the likelihood of becoming pregnant, prevention messages that focus on condom use are in direct conflict with this value (*Advocates for Youth, 1994*). Moreover, mistrust of western medical practices can make the use of birth control methods administered through clinical settings unlikely. The African American community welcomes and cares for children regardless of the age or marital status of parents and tends to be more accepting of sexual activity outside of marriage than other cultural groups (*Johnson, 1994*).

Latinas have the highest teen birth rate among the major racial/ethnic groups in the United States. Whereas overall two out of five young women in the U.S. get pregnant by age 20, three out of five young Hispanic women get pregnant at least once by age 20 (*The National Campaign to Prevent Teen Pregnancy, 2001*). Among traditional Latinas, "good girls" are sexually naive. Consequently, being prepared for sexual experiences by discussing intimacy or having a condom might not be considered appropriate (*Johnson, 1994*). Moreover, condom use is perceived by Latino men as unmanly and an obstacle to intimacy and control of sexual relations. Religion also plays a tremendous role. For example, over 85% of Latinos are Catholic. Consequently, the Catholic ban on contraceptive use makes it difficult to persuade Catholic Latinos to use condoms (*Advocates for Youth, 1994*).

Safer sex practices require that partners talk to one another about sexual histories, condom use, boundaries, etc. Because in most Latino/Latina families, discussions of sex are taboo, Latino/Latina students may never have talked about sexuality-related topics in public before. These conversations are difficult for almost everyone but among Latinos/Latinas, talking directly about sex in public or private is essentially unacceptable. Consequently, talk about sexual subjects may startle or offend these students and their families.

Language can be a barrier in almost every classroom. Colloquial or slang terms might distress or embarrass students who have been taught that certain words are offensive, or confuse those who are unfamiliar with them. On the other hand, some people prefer language that communicates what is felt, which may not be considered "proper English" (*Johnson, 1994*). School personnel need to be sensitive to the fact that young people may feel some conflict between what they are taught at home and what is being discussed. School personnel need to be aware of their own values and not seek to impose them upon classroom participants. Creating a safe environment and establishing trust are essential for discussing the personal issues associated with sexuality.

In working with African American youth, school personnel need to be sensitive to research observations demonstrating that teachers tend to demand less of African American youth, call on them less frequently, praise them less often, and give them less time to answer. Program activities that are effective with this population include storytelling, music, role-playing, African-American literature, debate, group learning, and games that build on cooperation.

Five key concepts for cultural competence proposed by one author (*Johnson, 1994*) can apply to any successful school sexuality program:

* Understand the values of the families and communities of which students are a part.

* For younger teens, focus on delaying the onset of sexual activity. For older teens, focus on preventing pregnancy through

Activities for Meeting the Challenge of Culturally Diverse Classrooms

Cultural competence involves providing students with engaging, effective programs; speaking to their cultural experience; reinforcing positive health messages received at home; and helping students be comfortable with their racial and ethnic identities and sexual orientation. Activities for achieving these include:

* Incorporating traditional cultural elements that reinforce the attitudes and skills you are seeking to develop.

* Inviting men and women who share students' cultural backgrounds to speak or volunteer in the school.

* Assuming that a wide range of views, particularly about sexuality issues, exists among your students. Demonstrate a willingness to listen to ideas that differ from yours.

* Getting to know students as individuals, not regarding them solely as representatives of an ethnic or racial group.

* Involving family members in program planning and activities.

* Using activities, discussions, videos, written materials, and guest speakers that reflect the cultural and ethnic diversity of the students, the community, and society in general.

* In a class representing diverse cultures and backgrounds, grouping students in mixed teams or partnerships working toward a common goal.

* Recognizing the cultural roots of students' behaviors. Don't expect all students to behave the same.

* Supporting students' exploration of their ethnic and racial identities.

* Engaging students in ongoing dialogues about stereotypes and the limits imposed by them.

* Seeking multicultural training for oneself and continue the process of building one's own cultural competence.

—Adapted from Advocates for Youth, 1994

contraceptive use.

* Document and address common myths related to sexuality.

* Develop programs to help young adults identify realistic, alternative life goals that will override the notion that pregnancy increases one's status or gains commitment from a partner.

* Work cooperatively with other community professionals such as clergy and youth leaders to deliver consistent messages.

Sexual Assault

Sexual assault (or "sexual abuse") refers to unwanted sexual acts, ranging from exhibitionism to penetration, that involve threats, physical force, intimidation, or deception. Sexual assault is often referred to as "childhood sexual abuse" when there is a significant (5 or more years) age difference between the individuals involved. Various forms of sexual assault are also referred to as "rape." This includes attempted or completed nonconsensual sexual acts committed by a person unknown to the victim (stranger rape), acts committed by someone known to the victim (acquaintance rape), acts committed within a dating relationship (date rape), acts committed in the context of a marriage or intimate live-in partnership (marital rape), acts committed by a family member (incest), and acts committed by two or more people (gang rape) (*American College of Obstetricians and Gynecologists, 2000*).

Children and adolescents who have been sexually assaulted are at increased risk for pregnancy, HIV infection, STDs and other negative outcomes. Unfortunately, the personal skills needed to prevent pregnancy are precisely those that are eradicated by sexual abuse. One quarter of pregnant and parenting adolescents are victims of partner abuse, and as many as two-thirds were abused as children. Victims of abuse and interpersonal violence are often unable to negotiate their sexual behaviors. Without the necessary skills and healing support, victimization and coercive sexual relationships are likely to continue *(Center for Assessment and Policy Development & National Organization on Adolescent Pregnancy, Parenting and Prevention, 2001)*. For these reasons, school personnel must be aware of the connection between teen pregnancy and sexual abuse and work to include assault prevention as a component in any teen pregnancy prevention strategy *(Advocates for Youth, 1995)*.

Childhood Sexual Abuse

Child sexual abuse occurs among all ethnic, racial, and socio-economic groups and in rural, suburban, and urban areas. One study on the prevalence of child sexual abuse found that 27% of women and 16% of men reported abuse. Children are most vulnerable between ages 8-12. Most are abused by someone they know and trust, although boys are more likely than girls to be abused by someone outside the family. Abuse typically occurs within a long-term relationship that escalates over time.

"By the time a student reaches middle school, he or she may have already learned what it's like to have been a victim of or witness to bullying, harassment, and even physical and sexual abuse. Similarly, students and staff need to have some sense of the scope and impact of sexual assault because such information can potentially reduce victim isolation and stress the importance of reducing the problem."

"It is vital for instructors, staff, and students to realize that the impact of such violence is felt across a broad spectrum of society. Health, mental health, substance abuse, and criminal justice systems find themselves providing services to those who have been victimized. And the community as a whole struggles with a variety of what are commonly referred to as 'social problems,' such as homelessness and teen pregnancy that seem to be, in part, a response to the impact of abuse over the lifespan."

—The American College of Obstetricians and Gynecologists, no date

In up to 50% of reported cases, offenders are adolescents (*Advocates for Youth, 1995*).

Sometimes victims of sexual abuse exhibit sexually provocative behavior or act out sexually in other ways. Survivors of child and adolescent sexual abuse experience a range of disorders, such as depression, substance abuse, eating disorders, sexual revictimization, anxiety, fear, hostility, chronic tension, low self-esteem, self-destructive or suicidal behavior, running away, criminal behavior, academic problems, prostitution, or other interpersonal and social difficulties. Teachers, coaches, nurses, bus drivers, and other school personnel are in an excellent position to recognize behaviors that might indicate that something is wrong. For example, a good student may suddenly score low on tests, refuse to change for gym, or keep missing the school bus. When school personnel notice suspicious signs, they are required by law to report what they observe to child protective services agencies. In fact, school employees have been responsible for identifying more than half of all children reported to be experiencing abuse or neglect (*Advocates for Youth, 1995; National Education Association, no date; Sechrist, 2000; Washington State Department of Health, 1999*).

Sometimes students will tell a favorite teacher or some other school staff person whom they trust that they have been abused. In planning for this possibility, school personnel need to be aware of the procedures for responding to disclosures of abuse in their jurisdiction and be prepared to offer one of the following recommended responses (*American College of Obstetricians and Gynecologists, 2000*):

* "It took a lot of courage for you to tell me this."

* "What happened to you is not your fault."

* "You don't deserve to be treated this way."

* "You're not alone and you're not crazy. Violence in families, in relationships, and among people who are acquainted is more common than you think."

Risk Factors for Sexual Victimization

* Girls who have few friends, absent or unavailable parents, a stepfather, and conflict with or between parents

* Physical or mental disability

* Separate living arrangements from both biological parents

* Mental illness or alcohol or drug abuse in the family

* A parent who was physically or sexually abused as a child

* Homes with other forms of abuse, prostitution, or transient adults

* Being a gay or lesbian youth

—Advocates for Youth, 1995.

NEA, as part of its Safe Schools efforts, supports efforts to prevent child abuse. These include employee awareness programs that provide information on identification of and reporting procedures for maltreated children. Teaching about child abuse in the classroom can contribute to finding help for children. For example, some students might have siblings or friends who are being abused. Following a discussion about abuse, a teacher might say: "If

this is happening to you, or to your brother or sister or a friend, please see me so we can talk about it." This could lead to two positive outcomes: someone can intervene to end the abuse and the abused child could receive professional services to begin the healing process (*Sechrist, 2000*).

Date Rape

Over half of all students in public secondary schools want to know more about what to do in cases of rape or sexual assault (*Kaiser Foundation, 2000a*). An estimated 60% of adolescents who have sex before age 15 do so involuntarily (*Alan Guttmacher Institute, 1994*). In a study that followed a cohort of young women from grades 8 to 12, almost one in four participants reported sexual coercion by dates or boyfriends. Female teens cite pressure from a boyfriend, the desire to please or keep a boyfriend, or feeling unable to say "no" as reasons for participating in unwanted sexual activities.

Some cases of date rape probably occur because of faulty assumptions and poor communications. These assumptions include rigid views of male and female gender roles, acceptance of rape myths (such as the notion that women "want" to be raped), and general distrust between men and women. One survey found that two out of three students believe that a male is not at fault if he rapes a girl who dresses "provocatively" on a date. One quarter of those students thought it would not be rape if a male got

Warning Signs That a Child May Have Been Sexually Abused

* Fear of certain people or places, e.g., fear of male parent or guardian

* Resistance to being touched; wariness of physical contact, especially when initiated by an adult

* Seductive behavior for approval

* Apprehensiveness when other children cry

* Unexplained prolonged absence (guardian may keep child at home while injury heals)

* Sudden mood swings: rage, fear, anger, withdrawal

* An older child behaving like a younger child, such as bedwetting or thumbsucking

* Sexual activities with toys or other children, such as simulating sex with dolls or asking other children to behave sexually

* New words for body parts

* Refusing to talk about a "secret" he or she has with an adult or older child

* Talking about a new older friend

* Suddenly having money

* Cutting or burning himself or herself as an adolescent

* Sleep problems such as nightmares, trouble sleeping, fear of the dark

* Extreme fear of "monsters"

* Spacing out at odd times

* Loss of appetite; trouble eating or swallowing

* Stomach illness all of the time with no identifiable reason

From: American Academy of Pediatrics
http://www.aap.org and
Stop It Now, http://www.stopitnow.org

his date drunk and had sex with her after she had said "no" to sexual intercourse. Prevention programs can address attitudes such as these by:

* discussing cultural beliefs about power, sexuality, and violence

* stressing that boys and men, not girls and women, are primarily responsible for preventing sexual assault

* recognizing that boys and men, as well as girls and women, can be victims of sexual assault

* promoting healthy relationship skills by helping youth distinguish between appropriate and inappropriate interpersonal behavior; boys and men learn alternative, nonviolent ways to express their masculinity; and girls and women learn to assert themselves and communicate their needs

* showing boys and girls how to support victims and respond to sexually aggressive behavior when this behavior is directed at someone else

(*American College of Obstetricians and Gynecologists, no date*)

Sample Abuse Reporting Policy

Any employee employed by the school district, including administrators, teachers, counselors, social workers, nurses, psychologists, bus drivers, educational assistants, child development technicians, or other agents of the district, shall report suspected cases of child abuse and child neglect to the local welfare agency, police department, or the county sheriff. All reporters must also simultaneously report cases of child abuse to the building principal. The building principal will be responsible to make all follow-up reports to the district office.

Definition of sexual abuse: Sexual abuse includes rape, sodomy, sexual intercourse with a child, indecent liberties, prostitution, and pornography. Indecent liberties include the intentional touching of the victim's intimate parts (genital area, groin, inner thigh, buttocks, or breast), or the coerced touch by the victim of an adult's intimate parts. Allegations of these actions must be reported to an investigative agency.

NOTE: Sexual abuse does not include hugging, kissing, pinching, or other touching if there is no touching of intimate parts as defined above. Although these actions may not be appropriate in some situations and may require administrative involvement, they need not be reported to an investigative agency as abuse.

—Excerpt from Minneapolis Public Schools

Successful programs are comprehensive; feature intensive, long-term, and interactive teaching approaches; are relevant to students; and contain positive messages about healthy relationships and what can be done for people who have experienced sexual assault. They should:

* inform participants about relevant school policies and local, state, and federal policies and laws

* examine what is meant by "consent" and communicate that sexual activity is a choice

* explore how alcohol and other drugs contribute to aggressive behavior and personal vulnerability by diminishing self control and decision-making ability

* teach students to analyze and interpret media messages that reinforce gender stereotypes and display inappropriate portrayals of power and sexuality

Appropriate sexuality education can help students understand the difference between a healthy and unhealthy relationship and develop the communication skills to clearly articulate their feelings and decisions. Educational opportunities in which young men and women learn to understand their desires and limits are important. Promoting self-discipline and respect for others is another important set of principles students need to learn. In Polk County, Florida students in grades 9-10 learn about conditions that may contribute to date rape and strategies for protection. The district recommends that a professional in the field of sexual assault teach this lesson. In twelfth grade, students learn about warning signs or "red flags" that may indicate a tendency for date rape. This lesson is intended to help students recognize strategies that might help prevent date rape as well as eliminate common myths and feelings of guilt.

Sexual Harassment

Sexual harassment is unwelcome intimidating, hostile, or offensive sexual behavior that interferes with one's daily activities. Sexual harassment can be a way that one person tries to make another vulnerable by behaving in a way that is inappropriate and unacceptable. This behavior can be in the form of language, touching, or other conduct (*U.S. Department of Education Office of Civil Rights, 1999*). Examples include sexual comments, jokes and gestures, requests for sexual favors, spreading sexual rumors about an individual, sexual advances, and an administrator's or supervisor's failure to prevent a hostile environment (*American College of Obstetricians and Gynecologists, 2000*). At school, sexual harassment can happen between students, or between staff, or between staff and students. Gay and lesbian youth are particularly vulnerable *(Jones, 1999)*.

Schools need to have policies that address sexual harassment, including a clear, easily available procedure for investigating and dealing with an allegation and appropriate measures to prevent further harassment in the school setting. Outside experts such as attorneys or social service professionals can educate staff, students, and families about

* laws relating to sexual harassment in schools
* community notification statutes
* confidentiality laws and policies
* relevant state statutes
* professional codes of conduct

Students, parents and school staff need to have open discussions about which behaviors are inappropriate and how to avoid or stop them. Individuals have different personal boundaries and ideas regarding what is acceptable in an educational setting. Consequently, these boundaries are not always clear. The lack of clarity makes it important for students and staff to discuss scenarios openly and flesh out what should and should not be tolerated. Students need to know that, if they feel that they are being sexually harassed, they should report their concern to a trusted parent, teacher, school counselor, or administrator.

Resources for Building Cultural Competence

Youth Leader's Guide to Building Cultural Competence, available from Advocates for Youth (Phone: (202) 347-5700: Website: http://www.advocatesforyouth.org), addresses providing HIV/STD and sexuality

Questions to ask regarding sexual harassment in your district or school:

* Does my school or district have a specific policy against harassment and a written code of conduct that publicizes it?

* Does the policy address sexual, racial/ethnic, sexual orientation, and differently-abled harassment?

* Does the policy contain the minimum elements of a definition, procedures, sanctions, and methods for notifying people?

* Is there a procedure to inform new employees and students about the policy?

* Is there reference to harassment in the student discipline code?

* Does the student handbook contain policy language regarding harassment?

* Do union contracts and affirmative action plans for the district contain policy language regarding harassment?

* Is there a grievance procedure that has been disseminated to staff and students and included in union contracts?

* Are there trained complaint managers who work cooperatively with administrators to apply sanctions and remedies and maintain regular reports regarding complaints filed and their disposition?

* Have students and staff been sensitized to the issue of harassment?

—Adapted from Larson, 1999

education to culturally diverse groups. This resource aims to build attitudes, knowledge, and skills necessary to reach all groups of young people with a focus on African American, Latino, and lesbian, gay, and bisexual teens.

The Spirit of Culture: Applying Cultural Competency to Strength-based Youth Development aims to make the Search Institute's assets approach "culturally inclusive, relevant across ethnicities and respectful of diverse approaches toward nurturing a child." This 52-page publication contains essays examining personal cultural identity as well as worksheets and training materials to use in cultural competency workshops. Available for $20 from Assets for Colorado Youth, *http://www.buildassets.org*.

Resources for Addressing Sexual Assault Prevention

Interpersonal Violence and Adolescent Pregnancy: Prevalence and Implications for Practice and Policy, developed by the Center for Assessment and Policy Development and the National Organization on Adolescent Pregnancy, Parenting, and Prevention, Inc., (NOAPPP), discusses the links between inter-personal violence and teen pregnancy, opportunities and challenges for policy development, and possible next steps for the field. The full-text is available on The Healthy Teen Network's (formerly NOAPPP) website: *http://www.healthyteennetwork.org*.

Unequal Partners: Teaching About Power and Consent in Adult-Teen Relationships is available from *Planned Parenthood of Greater Northern New Jersey, 196 Speedwell Avenue, Morristown, NJ 07960.*
Phone: (973) 539-9580, ext. 120.
Website: http://www.ppgnnj.org

This manual is designed to help professionals educate young people to make healthy decisions about relationships, especially those involving the power imbalances that can occur when there are significant age differences. The 24 interactive lessons help young people ages 10-17:

* identify characteristics of relationships which are honest, equal, and responsible

* rehearse skills for asserting their relationship rights

* practice responding to a variety of situations regarding unhealthy relationships

* examine legal issues, including age of consent, in their own state

* know the particular risks and issues

regarding adult-teen relationships.

Although the goal is to confront the issue of teen female-adult male relationships, some exercises are applicable to other relationships as well, including teen male-adult female and same sex relationships.

The American Psychological Association has developed a brochure for students called "***Love Doesn't Have to Hurt Teens***," available at *http://www.apa.org/pi/pii/teen*

How to Prevent Date Rape-Teen Tips, available from Advocates for Youth, gives suggestions for avoiding dangerous situations. For more information, go to:
http://www.advocatesforyouth.org

Resources for Addressing Harassment

Information about harassment, sample policies, and procedures for implementing policies in schools can be found in ***Protecting Students from Harassment and Hate Crime: A Guide for Schools***, available from the U.S. Department of Education Office for Civil Rights at *http://www.ed.gov/about/offices/list/ocr.*

Every state department of education has an equal education opportunity office that may have information on curriculum guides, workshops, videos, and other resources related to sexual harassment.

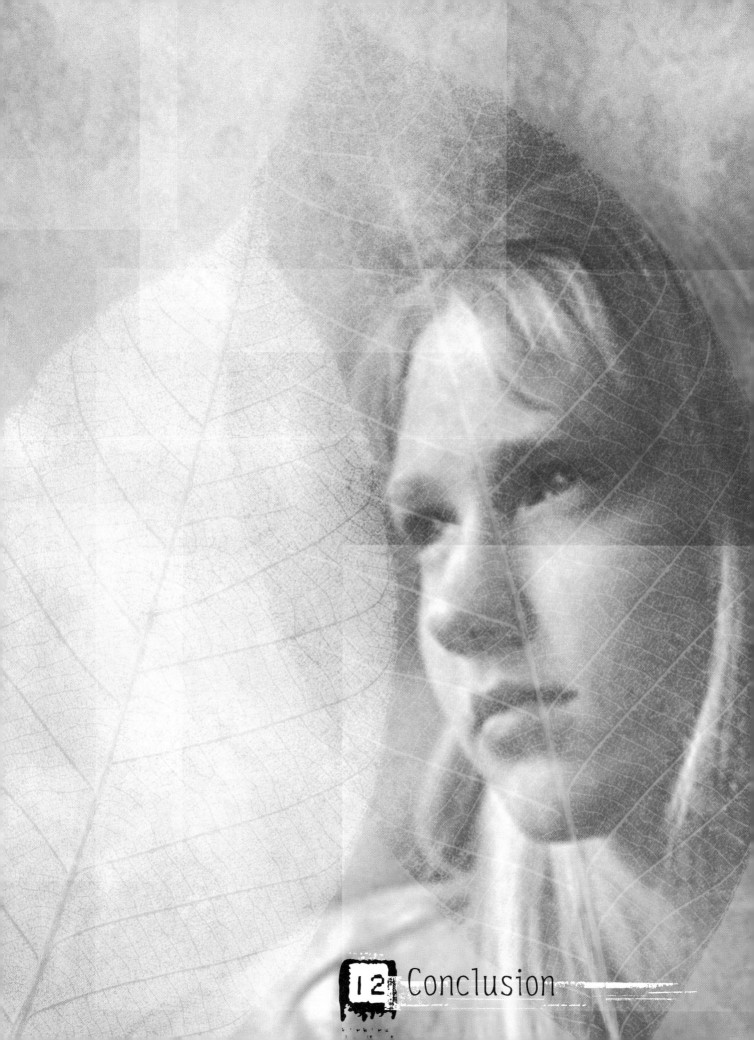

12 Conclusion

Teen pregnancy is

a deeply rooted social phenomenon that will continue to challenge society for years to come, despite promising recent declines. Its origins are tied to a number of other issues which collectively threaten the health and academic success of young men and women. Schools are in a unique position to reduce that threat. They have daily access to a captive audience of young people and are filled with professionals who care deeply about children and are trained to develop the success and potential of each student.

This publication was designed to help school personnel understand and discover the opportunities they have to promote teen pregnancy prevention and sexual responsibility among school-aged youth. Indeed, the support of schools is invaluable. The NEA's hope is that the information and suggestions contained in this document will better prepare educators, support professionals, and other school personnel to carry out their role in promoting the health and success of every student.

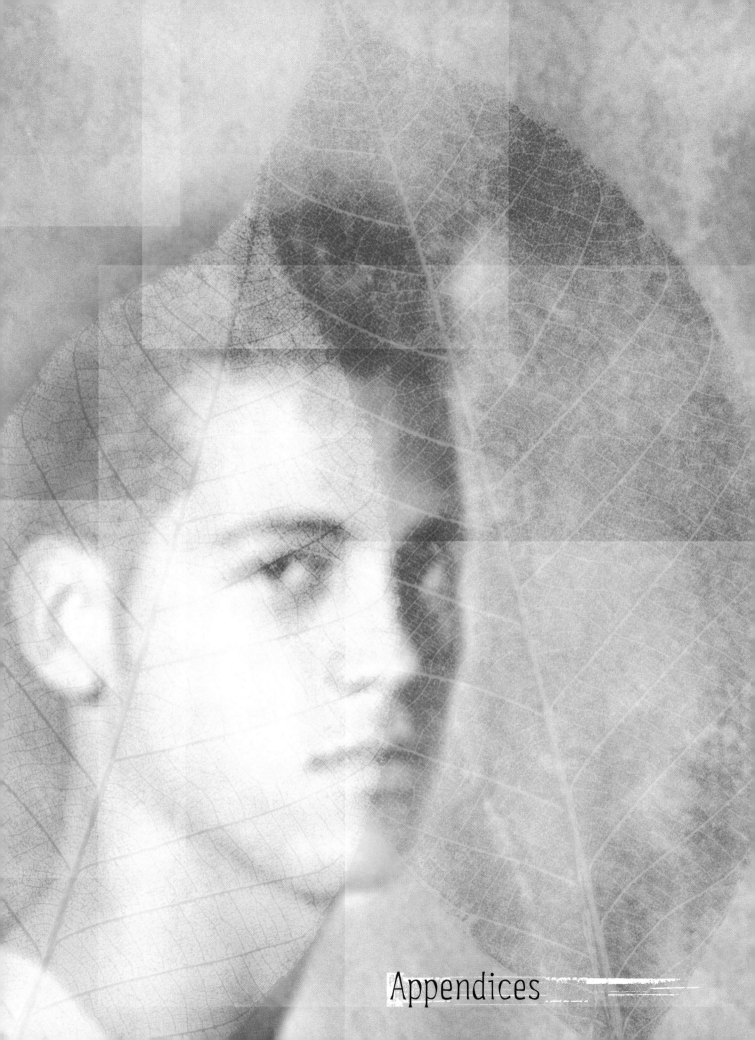

Appendices

Appendix A

National Organizations and Websites that Address Teen Pregnancy Prevention

Disclaimer: Listing national organizations and websites does not imply endorsement of their content.

Advocates for Youth

2000 M Street, N.W., Suite 750

Washington, DC 20036

Phone: (202) 419-3420

Website: *http://www.advocatesforyouth.org*

Works to increase the opportunities and abilities of youth to make healthy decisions about sexuality by providing information, education, and advocacy. Published *Communities Responding to the Challenge of Adolescent Pregnancy Prevention*, a five-volume series that outlines strategies for reaching youth at risk for early pregnancy, and numerous fact sheets as well as items mentioned throughout this document.

The Alan Guttmacher Institute

120 Wall Street

New York, NY 10005

Phone: (212) 248-1111

Website: *http://www.agi-usa.org*

A not-for-profit organization for sexual and reproductive health research, policy analysis, and public education. Their website is full of up-to-date statistics and fact sheets on a range of issues related to women's and men's health in the U.S. and internationally.

American Alliance for Health, Physical Education, Recreation and Dance (AAHPERD)

1900 Association Drive

Reston, VA 20191-1599

Phone: (703) 476-3400

Website: *http://www.aahperd.org*

AAHPERD has regional and state-level affiliates that work to promote the health of young people in their area. To identify the affiliate in a state, go to the AAHPERD website, click on "districts" and then find the state.

American Association of School Administrators

1801 N. Quincy Street, Suite 700

Arlington, VA 22203

Phone: (703) 528-0700

Website: *http://www.aasa.org*

American Cancer Society

Website: *http://www.cancer.org*

Local divisions may have information about state coalitions that address promoting the health of young people in school.

American Social Health Association

Phone: (919) 361-8400

Website: *http://www.ashastd.org*

ASHA is a nonprofit organization dedicated to stopping sexually transmitted diseases and their harmful consequences among individuals, families, and communities. The website offers information on sexually transmitted diseases, names of support groups for STDs, glossary of sexual health terms, list of STD hotlines, and a website for youth (*www.iwannaknow.org*) that offers advice and information about topics such as peer pressure, puberty, abstinence, love and sex, STDs, and date rape. There is also a chat room where teens can talk to one another about sexuality.

Centers for Disease Control and Prevention Division of Sexually Transmitted Diseases

Phone: (1-800) 227-8922

Website: *http://www.cdc.gov/std/*

The website offers statistics on STDs, guidelines for treatment, list of STD hotlines, and list of publications concerning STDs.

ETR Associates

Maintains **ReCAPP** (Resource Center for Adolescent Pregnancy Prevention), (*http://www.etr.org/recapp*) a website that provides regularly updated information on programs, practices, and resources. Numerous curricula, publications, and other relevant materials are available from ETR Associates

P.O. Box 1830, Santa Cruz, CA 95061

Phone: 831-438-4060

Website: *http://www.etr.org*

Kaiser Family Foundation

Phone: (650) 854-9400

Website: *http://www.kff.org*

The website offers information on adolescent sexual health, sex education, contraception, STDs, unintended pregnancy, and other sexual health information.

The National Campaign to Prevent Teen Pregnancy

1776 Massachusetts Avenue, N.W., Suite 200

Washington, DC 20036

Phone: (202) 478-8500

Website: *http://www.teenpregnancy.org*

Published *Get Organized: A Guide to Preventing Teenage Pregnancy* as well as many other useful documents. The website offers up-to-date facts and statistics on teen pregnancy; publications for a range of different audiences including communities, faith leaders, parents and teens (English and Spanish versions); information specifically for teens; and press releases and legislative updates.

National 4-H Council

Website: *http://www.bpy.n4h.org*

Sponsors "Building Partnerships for Youth," a project that provides assistance to organizations and communities that choose to provide abstinence programming to youth ages 9 to 13 using a youth development approach.

Healthy Teen Network

Phone: (202) 547-8814

Website: *http://www.healthyteennetwork.org*

Provides leadership on adolescent pregnancy prevention and adolescent parenting issues. Membership includes teachers and other school employees.

The National PTA

330 North Wabash Avenue, Suite 2100

Chicago, IL 60611

Phone: (312) 670-6782

Website (*http://www.pta.org*) offers pamphlets on *Talking With Your Child About Sex* and *Talking With Your Teen About Sex.*

National Youth Advisory Coalition
Planned Parenthood Federation of America

Phone: (212) 541-7800

Website: *http://www.plannedparenthood.org*

The website offers pamphlets on family communication, abstinence, teen sexuality, STDs, contraception, pregnancy, and general health issues. These are tailored for different audiences, including parents, teens, women, men, and health providers. The website also offers advice on parenting and pregnancy.

The Search Institute

625 Fourth Avenue So.

Minneapolis, MN 55415

Phone: (800) 888-3820

Website: *http://www.search-institute.org*

Provides information and materials on youth development including youth needs assessment surveys and reports that connect assets to behavioral choices. Developed *Values and Choices* curriculum.

Sexuality Information and Education Council of the United States (SIECUS)

130 West 42nd Street, Suite 35

New York, NY 10019

Phone: (212) 819-9770

Website: *http://www.siecus.org*

Provides information on sexuality for educators and parents. Publishes *Guidelines for Comprehensive Sexuality Education, Kindergarten-12th Grade* and other materials relating to young people's sexual health. *Filling the Gaps: Hard to Teach Topics in Sexuality Education* provides background information, reasons for teaching each topic, and classroom activities. It addresses abstinence, teaching condom use, pregnancy options, safer sex, sexual orientation, sexual health, and an appreciation of diversity. The website offers tips for parents on how to talk to kids about sex, sexuality information for teens, sexual education curriculum for faith institutions, over 50 publications on sexual health issues, and a radio series on Frequently Asked Questions.

Appendix B
Checklist and Charts

Teen Pregnancy Prevention Checklist—Use the checklist to determine what is in place and to plan future activities.

Chart I: Inventory of School and Community Programs, Activities, and Policies to Prevent Teen Pregnancy—Use this chart to identify gaps, overlaps, duplications, and potential for collaboration by listing current activities and the components that address them.

Chart II: How We Can Support Teen Pregnancy Prevention (or Who Will Support Teen Pregnancy Prevention)—Use this chart to identify how each component can support teen pregnancy prevention. Add other squares such as students or teachers, if desired.

Chart III: Community Action Plan—Use this form to plan your activities.

Chart IV: Current Funding for Teen Pregnancy Prevention in My Community—Use this form to identify all the funding sources that support teen pregnancy prevention activities and then look for opportunities to share.

Teen Pregnancy Prevention Checklist

KEY

<ul>
<li>☐ 1 *Does not exist*</li>
<li>☐ 2 *Under development*</li>
<li>☐ 3 *In place*</li>
</ul>

POLICIES

My school has policies that:

* promote a healthy environment   ☐1 ☐2 ☐3

* support a K-12 sexuality education program within the context of a coordinated school health program   ☐1 ☐2 ☐3

* require training for teachers and other school personnel   ☐1 ☐2 ☐3

* promote family involvement   ☐1 ☐2 ☐3

* define and present procedures for addressing sexual harassment   ☐1 ☐2 ☐3

* provide for reporting suspected sexual abuse   ☐1 ☐2 ☐3

* protect the confidentiality of students and staff   ☐1 ☐2 ☐3

* address the treatment of pregnant and parenting teens   ☐1 ☐2 ☐3

CLASSROOM

The district/school has a scope and sequence for a K-12 health education program that includes sexuality education.   ☐1 ☐2 ☐3

Sexuality education curricula are research-based, evaluated, and found to be effective.   ☐1 ☐2 ☐3

Teachers are trained to teach the program and receive booster sessions on a regular basis.   ☐1 ☐2 ☐3

Prevention messages and health facts are integrated into other academic areas.   ☐1 ☐2 ☐3

School staff understand the sexuality education program and reinforce classroom learning in conversations and by setting examples.   ☐1 ☐2 ☐3

The media center has materials that reinforce classroom learning.   ☐1 ☐2 ☐3

SERVICES

Teachers and staff are aware of services available to students and their families.   ☐1 ☐2 ☐3

Teachers and staff know how to identify students who might need to be referred for services.   ☐1 ☐2 ☐3

Teachers and staff know how to respond when students share problems with them.   ☐1 ☐2 ☐3

The school/district has a well-defined referral process.   ☐1 ☐2 ☐3

Teachers and staff understand the referral process, including issues related to confidentiality.   ☐1 ☐2 ☐3

Teen Pregnancy Prevention Checklist (continued)

KEY

1. *Does not exist*
2. *Under development*
3. *In place*

SPECIAL POPULATIONS

My school/district is prepared to address the unique needs of:

* Pregnant and parenting teens ☐1 ☐2 ☐3

* Students with special needs ☐1 ☐2 ☐3

* Young males ☐1 ☐2 ☐3

* Gay, lesbian, bisexual, trans-gender, and questioning youth ☐1 ☐2 ☐3

* Sexually-abused students ☐1 ☐2 ☐3

* Diverse cultures ☐1 ☐2 ☐3

STRUCTURE

Administrators and policy makers understand and support activities to address sexuality and teen pregnancy prevention. ☐1 ☐2 ☐3

A representative school health advisory committee or teen pregnancy prevention committee meets regularly. ☐1 ☐2 ☐3

An individual has been designated to coordinate school health and teen pregnancy prevention activities. ☐1 ☐2 ☐3

A community coalition that includes parents, students, businesses, community agencies and organizations, faith leadership, and other interested citizens provides a forum for community opinions and rallies support for activities. ☐1 ☐2 ☐3

PLANNING

Data have been gathered to inform program planning including relevant national, state, and local policies; the incidence of STDs and teen pregnancy in the community; an inventory of resources that currently address these issues; and an assessment of school staff, family, student, and community understanding and support. ☐1 ☐2 ☐3

A plan with realistic goals, measurable objectives, steps to achieve these objectives, designated responsibility, identified resources, timeline, and monitoring and evaluation procedures has been developed. ☐1 ☐2 ☐3

STAFF DEVELOPMENT

Staff development is offered regularly to ensure that all teachers and staff understand policies and programs. ☐1 ☐2 ☐3

New teachers and staff receive orientation so that all staff have the same understanding. ☐1 ☐2 ☐3

Teen Pregnancy Prevention Checklist (continued)

KEY

1. *Does not exist*
2. *Under development*
3. *In place*

COMMUNICATIONS

All stakeholders, including administrators, school staff, students, parents, and the community are informed regularly about program activities, status, and impact, using strategies such as:

* regular reports to administrators and the school board   1 2 3

* messages and updates included regularly in district and school newsletters   1 2 3

* articles and features in local newspapers and other media   1 2 3

* displays in schools and the community   1 2 3

* health fairs   1 2 3

* events during Teen Pregnancy Prevention month   1 2 3

* other _____   1 2 3

* _____

   _____   1 2 3

OTHER ACTIVITIES THAT SUPPORT YOUTH DEVELOPMENT AND HEALTHY SEXUALITY

After-school programs   1 2 3

Peer support groups   1 2 3

Peer teaching, e.g., high school students meeting with younger students   1 2 3

Other_____   1 2 3

CHART I

Inventory of School and Community Programs, Activities, and Policies to Prevent Teen Pregnancy

Activity, Program, or Policy	Coordinated School Health Program Component								
	HED	PE	HS	NS	HPS	CPSS	HSE	FCI

HED=health education, PE=physical education, HS=health services, NS=nutrition services, HPS=health promotion for staff (staff wellness), CPSS=counseling, psychological, and social services, HSE=healthy school environment, FCI=family and community involvement

Source: Adapted from *Talking About Health is Academic*, Teachers College Press.

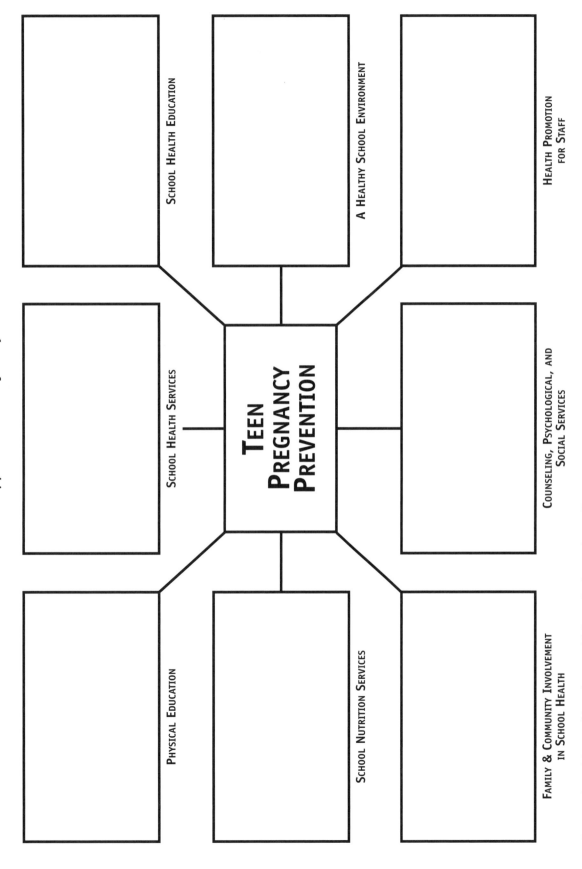

CHART II

How We Can Support Teen Pregnancy Prevention

SCHOOL HEALTH EDUCATION

A HEALTHY SCHOOL ENVIRONMENT

HEALTH PROMOTION FOR STAFF

SCHOOL HEALTH SERVICES

TEEN PREGNANCY PREVENTION

COUNSELING, PSYCHOLOGICAL, AND SOCIAL SERVICES

PHYSICAL EDUCATION

SCHOOL NUTRITION SERVICES

FAMILY & COMMUNITY INVOLVEMENT IN SCHOOL HEALTH

Source: Adapted from *Talking About Health is Academic,* Teachers College Press.

CHART III
Community Action Plan

GOAL: _____

OBJECTIVE: _____

ACTIVITY	PERSON(S) RESPONSIBLE	DATE COMPLETED	RESOURCES NEEDED

MAKE AS MANY COPIES OF THIS SHEET AS NEEDED

CHART IV

Current Funding for Teen Pregnancy in My Community

Coordinated School Health Program Component

Funding Source and $ amount	HED	PE	HS	NS	HPS	CPSS	HSE	FCI
Federal Sources								
State Sources								
Local Sources								
Other Sources								
Total Funding Available for Teen Pregnancy Activities								

HED=health education, PE=physical education, HS=health services, NS=nutrition services, HPS=health promotion for staff (staff wellness), CPSS=counseling, psychological, and social services, HSE=healthy school environment, FCI=family and community involvement

Source: Adapted from *Talking About Health is Academic*, Teachers College Press.

Appendix C
References

Advocates for Youth. (1994). *Youth Leader's Guide to Cultural Competence.* Washington, DC: Author.

Advocates for Youth. (1995). Child sexual abuse I: An overview. Washington, DC: Author. Online: http://www.advocatesfory-outh.org/factsheet/FSABUSE1.HTM

Advocates for Youth. (1997). School Condom Availability Fact Sheet. Washington, DC: Author.

Advocates for Youth. (2003). GLBTQ Youth: At Risk and Underserved Fact Sheet. Washington, DC: Author.

The Alan Guttmacher Institute. (1994). *Sex and America's Teenagers.* New York, NY: Author.

The Alan Guttmacher Institute. (1997). Teenagers' right to consent to reproductive health care. *Issues in Brief.* New York: Author.

The Alan Guttmacher Institute. (1998). Contraceptive use. *Facts In Brief.* New York: Author.

The Alan Guttmacher Institute. (2000). Trend toward abstinence-only sex ed means many U.S. teenagers are not getting vital messages about contraception. New York: Author. Online: http://www.agi-usa.org/pubs/archives/newsrelease3205.html

The Alan Guttmacher Institute. (2002). *Sexual and reproductive health: Women and men.* New York: Author.

Allen, J.P., Philliber, S., Herrling, S., & Kuperminc, G.P. (1997) Preventing teen pregnancy and academic failure: Experimental evaluation of a developmentally based approach. *Child Development,* 64:4, 729-742.

Allensworth, D.D. & Rubin, M. (1997). *A comprehensive approach to reduce pregnancy and the spread of HIV: An advocacy kit.* Kent, OH: American School Health Association.

American Academy of Pediatrics, Committee on Adolescence. (1995). Condom availability for youth. *Pediatrics,* 95:2, 281-285.

American College of Obstetricians and Gynecologists. (No date). *Drawing the line: A guide to developing effective sexual assault prevention programs for middle school students.* Washington, DC: Author.

Andersen, P. (2002). Health and science: Unintended consequences: Program precipitates drop in youth pregnancy rate. *Nando Times,* May 13. AP online. http://www.nan-dotimes.com/healthscience/story/400670p-3189736c.html

Bearman, P. & Bruckner, H. (1999). Peer effects on adolescent sexual debut and pregnancy: An analysis of a national survey of adolescent girls. In *Peer potential: Making the most of how teens influence each other*. Washington, DC: The National Campaign to Prevent Teen Pregnancy.

Bearman, P., Bruckner, H., Bradford, B., Theobald, W., & Philliber, S. (1999). *Peer potential: Making the most of how teens influence each other*. Washington, DC: National Campaign to Prevent Teen Pregnancy.

Becker, Robert. (1999). *Male involvement and adolescent pregnancy prevention*. Santa Cruz, CA: Resource Center for Adolescent Pregnancy Prevention, ETR Associates. Website: http://www.etr.org/recapp

Benson, P.L., Galbraith, J., & Espeland, P. (1998). *What kids need to succeed*. Minneapolis, MN: Free Spirit Publishing.

Black, S. (1998). Facts of life. *The American School Board Journal*, August 1998, pp. 33-36.

Blake, S.M., Ledsky, R., Goodenow, C., Sawyer, R., Lohrmann, D., & Windsor, R. (2003). Condom availability programs in Massachusetts high schools: Relationship with condom use and sexual behavior. *American Journal of Public Health*, 93(6), 955-962.

Blum, R.W. & Rinehart, P.M. (1997). *Reducing the risk: Connections that make a difference in the lives of youth*. Minneapolis, MN: University of Minnesota.

Blum, R.W., Beuhring, T., Shew, M.L., Bearinger, L.H., Sieving, R.E., & Resnick, M.D. (2000). The effects of race/ethnicity, income, and family structure on adolescent risk behaviors. *American Journal of Public Health*, 90:12, 1879-1884.

Blum, R.W., McNeely, C.A., & Rinehart, P.M. (2002). *Improving the odds: The untapped power of schools to improve the health of teens*. Minneapolis, MN: Center for Adolescent Health and Development, University of Minnesota.

Blumenfeld, W.J. (1994). Gay, lesbian, bisexual and questioning youth in *The sexuality education challenge: Promoting healthy sexuality in young people*, Judy C. Drolet and Kay Clark, eds. Santa Cruz, CA: ETR Associates.

Bogden, J.F., Fraser, K., Vega-Matos, C., & Ascroft, J. (1996). *Someone at school has AIDS: A complete guide to education policies concerning HIV infection*. Alexandria, VA: National Association of State Boards of Education.

Bogden, J. (2000). *Fit, healthy, and ready to learn: A school health policy guide*. Alexandria, VA: National Association of State Boards of Education.

Center for Assessment and Policy Development. (1999). *Providing services to all teen parents, both non-TANF and TANF*. Bala Cynwyd, PA: Author. Available at http://www.capd.org/home/services/teenparents/ta_adds/weblist12.pdf.

Center for Assessment and Policy Development. (1999). *Helping the education system work for teen parents and their children*. Bala Cynwyd, PA: Author.

Center for Assessment and Policy Development & National Organization on Adolescent Pregnancy, Parenting and Prevention. (2001). *Interpersonal violence and adolescent pregnancy: prevalence and implications for practice and policy*. Available on the internet at: http://www.healthyteennetwork.org

Centers for Schools and Communities. (1999). *A resource guide of best practices for pregnant and parenting teen programs*. Lemoyne, PA: Author.

Collins, J.L., Small, M.L., Kann, L., Pateman, B.C., Gold, R.S., & Kolbe, L.J. (1995). School health education. *Journal of School Health*, 65(8), 302-311.

Comprehensive Health Education Foundation. (1995). *Renewing the Partnership: The Mainline Church in Support of Public Education*. Seattle, WA: Author

Council of Chief State School Officers. (1999). *Teenage pregnancy: State education agencies and prevention*. Washington, DC: Author.

Council of Chief State School Officers. (March, 2000). How to tap TANF funding for extended learning programs. *Gaining Ground*. Available at http://www.ccsso.org.

Dailard, C. (2000). School-based health centers and the birth control debate. *The Guttmacher Report on Public Policy. Vol. 3, No. 5*. Available at http://www.agi-usa.org/pubs/ib_1200.html

Darroch, J.E., Landry, D.J., & Singh, S. (2000). Changing emphases in sexuality education in U.S. public secondary schools, 1988-1999. *Family Planning Perspectives*, 32(5), 204-211.

Devaney, B., Johnson, A., Maynard, R., & Trenholm, C. (2002). *The evaluation of abstinence education programs funded under Title V, Section 510: An interim report*. Princeton, NJ: Mathematica Policy Research Inc. Website: http://www.mathematica-mpr.com

Dryfoos, J.G. (1998). *Safe passages: Making it through adolescence in a risky society: What parents, schools, and communities can do*. New York: Oxford University Press.

Education Development Center. (1999). *Talking about Health Is Academic: Six workshop modules for promoting a coordinated approach to school health*. New York: Teachers College Press.

Flinn, S.K. & Hauser, D. (1998). *Teenage pregnancy: The case for prevention. An analysis of recent trends and federal expenditures associated with teenage pregnancy*. Washington, DC: Advocates for Youth.

Fetro, J.V. (1999). *Step by step to health-promoting schools*. Santa Cruz, CA: ETR Associates.

Garofalo, R., Wolf, C., Kessel, S., Palfrey, J., & Durant, R.H. (1998). The association between health risk behaviors and sexual orientation among a school-based sample of adolescents. *Pediatrics*, 101(5), 895-902.

The Gay, Lesbian, and Bisexual Speakers Bureau. (No date.) *How homophobia hurts us all*. Boston, MA: Author.

Gibson, P. (1989). *Gay male and lesbian youth suicide, Report of the Secretary's Task Force on Youth Suicide*. Washington, DC: U.S. Department of Health and Human Services.

Golonka, S., Lovejoy, A., & Stebbins, H. (2000). Serving children and youth through the Temporary Assistance for Needy Families Block Grant. Washington, DC: National Governors' Association Center. Available online: http://www.nga.org/Pubs/IssueBriefs/default.asp

Grunbaum, J.A., Kann, L.., Kinchen, S., Williams, B., Ross, J.G., Lowry, R., Kolbe, L. (2004). Youth risk behavior surveillance - United States, 2003. *Morbidity and Mortality Weekly Report*; June 21, 2004; 53(SS02). Available online: http://www.cdc.gov/HealthyYouth/yrbs/index.htm

Henshaw, S.K. (1998) Unintended pregnancy in the United States. *Family Planning Perspectives*, 30(1):24-29 & 46, Table 1.

Hurwitz, N. & Hurwitz, S. (2000) The case for school-based health centers. *American School Board Journal*, 187:24 August 2000.

Institute of Medicine. (1997). *Schools and health: Our nation's investment*. Washington, DC: National Academy Press.

Johnson, L.E. (1994). Cultural competence and sexuality education in *The sexuality challenge: Promoting healthy sexuality in young people*, (Drolet, J.C. & Clark, K., Eds.) Santa Cruz, CA: ETR Associates.

Jones, R. (1999). I don't feel safe here anymore. *American School Board Journal*, 186(11), 26-31.

Kaiser Family Foundation. (1999). *Kids & Media at the New Millennium*. Menlo Park, CA: Author

Kaiser Family Foundation/MTV/Teen People. (1999). *What teens know and don't (but should) about sexually transmitted diseases: A national survey of 15 to 17 year-olds.* Menlo Park, CA: Kaiser Family Foundation.

Kaiser Family Foundation. (2000a). *Sex education in America: A view from inside the nation's classrooms.* Menlo Park, CA: Author.

Kaiser Family Foundation. (2000b). Sex education in the U.S.: Policy and politics. *Issue Update*, September 2000. Menlo Park, CA: Author.

Kaiser Family Foundation. (2000c). *Decision making: A series of national surveys of teens about sex.* Menlo Park, CA: Author.

Kaiser Family Foundation. (2002). *Sex education in the U.S.: Policy and Politics.* Menlo Park, CA: Author.

Kaiser Family Foundation. (2003). *National Survey of Adolescents and Young Adults: Sexual Health Knowledge, Attitudes and Experiences.* Menlo Park, CA: Author.

Kalmuss, D.S. & Namerow, P.B. (1994). Subsequent childbearing among teenage mothers: The determinants of a closely spaced second birth. *Family Planning Perspectives*, 26(4): 149-153 & 159

Kelly, K.M., Vincent, M.L., Barnes, B., Lacson, R., & Rao, R. (no date). *Implementation standards and guidelines for community-based projects: Lessons learned from the school/community sexual risk reduction project.* Columbia, SC: University of South Carolina School of Public Health.

Kirby, D. (1997). *No easy answers: Research findings on programs to reduce teen pregnancy (Summary).* Washington, DC: The National Campaign to Prevent Teen Pregnancy.

Kirby, D. (2001). *Emerging answers: Research findings on programs to reduce teen pregnancy.* Washington, DC: National Campaign to Prevent Teen Pregnancy.

Klahn, J.K. & Iverson, C.J. (no date). *Roles for school nurses in adolescent pregnancy: Prevention, intervention, and support.* Lincoln, NE: Nebraska Department of Health.

Kunkel, D., Cope, K., Farinola, W., Biely, E., Rollin, E., & Donnerstein, E. (1999). *Sex on TV: Context and content.* Menlo Park, CA: Kaiser Family Foundation.

Landry, D.J., Kaeser, L., & Richards, C.L. (1999). Abstinence promotion and the provision of information about contraception in public school district sexuality education policies. *Family Planning Perspectives*, 31(6), 280-286.

Landry, D.J., Singh, S., & Darroch, J.E. (2000). Sexuality education in fifth and sixth grades in U.S. public schools. *Family Planning Perspectives*, 32(5), 212-219.

Larson, M. (1999). Checklist and survey: Is harassment a problem in your school? in *Protecting students from harassment and hate crime: A guide for schools.* Washington, DC: U.S. Department of Education Office for Civil Rights.

Lavin, A.T., Shapiro, G.R., & Weill, K.S. (1992). *Creating an agenda for school-based health promotion: A review of selected reports.* Boston, MA: Harvard School of Public Health.

Lonczak, H.S., Abbott, R.D., Hawkins, J.D., Kosterman, R., & Catalano, R. (2002). Effects of the Seattle social development project on sexual behavior, pregnancy, birth, and sexually transmitted disease outcomes by age 21 years. *Archives of Pediatrics and Adolescent Medicine,* 156 (5), 438-447.

Manlove, J. (1998). The influence of high school dropout and school disengagement on the risk of school-age pregnancy. *Journal of Research on Adolescence,* 8(2), 187-220.

Marx, E. & Northrop, D. (1995). *Educating for health: A guide to implementing a comprehensive approach to school health education.* Newton, MA: Education Development Center, Inc.

Marx, E., Wooley, S.F., & Northrop, D. (1998). *Health is academic: A guide to coordinated school health programs.* New York: Teachers College Press.

Maynard, R.A. (1996) *Kids having kids: A Robin Hood Foundation special report on the costs of adolescent childbearing.* New York, NY: Robin Hood Foundation.

Moore, K.A., Driscoll, A.K., & Ooms, T. (1997). *Not just for girls: The role of boys and men in teen pregnancy prevention.* Washington, DC: National Campaign to Prevent Teen Pregnancy.

Muccigrosso, Lynne. (1994). Special education students: Issues and needs in *The sexuality education challenge: Promoting healthy sexuality in young people.* (Judy C. Drolet and Kay Clark, eds.) Santa Cruz, CA: ETR Associates.

National Abortion and Reproductive Rights Action League (NARAL). (1998, 2003). *Who decides: A state by state review of abortion and reproductive rights.* Washington, DC: NARAL.

National Association of School Nurses. (2002). Frequently asked questions. Online: http://www.nasn.org.

National Assembly on School-Based Health Care. (2002). Data from school year 2001-02 census. Washington, DC: Author. Website: http://www.nasbhc.org/EQ/National_2001 Data.htm.

National Association of State Boards of Education. (1998). *Policy update: The role of education in teen pregnancy prevention.* Alexandria, VA: Policy Information Clearinghouse.

The National Campaign to Prevent Teen Pregnancy. (1997). *Whatever happened to childhood? The problem of teen pregnancy in the United States.* Washington, DC: Author.

The National Campaign to Prevent Teen Pregnancy. (1998a). *Start early, stay late: Linking youth development and teen pregnancy prevention.* Washington, DC: Author.

The National Campaign to Prevent Teen Pregnancy. (1998b) *Ten tips for parents to help their children avoid teen pregnancy.* Washington, DC: Author.

The National Campaign to Prevent Teen Pregnancy. (1999a). *Get organized: A guide to preventing teen pregnancy.* Washington, DC: Author.

The National Campaign to Prevent Teen Pregnancy. (1999b). *Are peers getting a bad rap? A 1999 poll.* Washington, DC: Author. On-line: http://www.teenpregnancy.org/poll4_99.pdf

The National Campaign to Prevent Teen Pregnancy. (1999c). *Talking back: Ten things teens want parents to know about teen pregnancy.* Washington, DC: Author.

The National Campaign to Prevent Teen Pregnancy. (1999d). *Nine tips to help faith leaders and their communities address teen pregnancy.* Washington, DC: Author.

The National Campaign to Prevent Teen Pregnancy. (2000). *Fact sheet: Why the education community should care about preventing teen pregnancy: Notes from the field.* Washington, DC: Author.

The National Campaign to Prevent Teen Pregnancy. (2000b). *Not just another thing to do: Teens tell us about sex, regret, and the influence of their parents.* Washington, DC: Author. On-line: http://www.teenpregnancy.org/teenwant.pdf

The National Campaign to Prevent Teen Pregnancy. (2000c). *Voices carry: Teens speak out on sex and teen pregnancy.* Washington, DC: Author.

The National Campaign to Prevent Teen Pregnancy. (2001). *Fact sheet: Teen sexual activity, pregnancy and childbearing among Latinos in the United States.* Washington, DC: Author.

The National Campaign to Prevent Teen Pregnancy. (2002) *Not just another single issue: Teen pregnancy prevention's link to other critical social issues.* Washington, DC: Author.

The National Campaign to Prevent Teen Pregnancy. (2004) *Just the facts: Powerpoint presentations on teen pregnancy and childbearing*. Washington, DC: Author.

The National Campaign to Prevent Teen Pregnancy. (2004) *With one voice: America's adults and teens sound off about teen pregnancy*. Washington, DC: Author.

The National Center on Addiction and Substance Abuse at Columbia. (1999). *Dangerous liaisons: Substance abuse and sex*. New York: The National Center on Addiction and Substance Abuse at Columbia.

National Coalition for Parent Involvement in Education. (no date). *Developing family/school partnerships: Guidelines for schools and school districts*. Washington, DC: Author. On-line: http://www.ncpieguide-lines.htm.

National Education Association. (No date). *Child abuse and neglect, Action Sheet*. Washington, DC: Author.

National Governors' Association. (2000). *Extra learning opportunities that encourage healthy lifestyles*. Washington, DC: Author. Website: http://www.nga.org/CBP/Activities/Extra Learning.asp

National Guidelines Task Force. (1996). *Guidelines for comprehensive sexuality education, 2nd edition*. New York: Sexuality Information and Education Council of the United States.

National School Boards Association. (1990). Reducing the risk: *A school leader's guide to AIDS education*. Alexandria, VA: Author.

National Task Force on Confidential Student Health Information, (2000). *Guidelines for protecting confidential student health information*. Kent, OH: American School Health Association.

Nickelodeon, Kaiser Family Foundation, & Children Now. (2001). *Talking with kids about tough issues: A national survey of parents and kids*. View at http://www.children-now.org/nickelodeon/summary.pdf

Parker-Pope, Tara. (2002). Abstinence gains unlikely ally in sex-education curriculum. *The Wall Street Journal*, August 27, D1.

The President's Council on Physical Fitness and Sports. (no date). *Physical activity and sport in the lives of girls: Physical and mental health dimensions from an interdisciplinary approach*. Washington, DC: Author.

Resource Center for Adolescent Pregnancy Prevention. (2000). *GLBYQ youth*. Santa Cruz, CA: ETR Associates. (http://www.etr.org/recapp)

Rotheram-Borus, M.J., Marelich, W.D., & Srinivasan, S. (1999). HIV risk among homosexual, bisexual, and heterosexual male and female youths. *Archives of Sexual Behavior*, 28(2), 159-176.

Ryan, C. & Futterman, D. (1998). *Lesbian and gay youth: Care and counseling*. New York: Columbia University Press.

Sabo, D., Miller, K., Farrell, M., Barnes, G., & Melnick, M. (1998). *The Women's Sports Foundation report: Sports and teen pregnancy*. East Meadow, NY: Women's Sports Foundation.

Saewyc, E.M., Bearinger, L.H., Blum, R.W., & Resnick (1998). Gender differences in health and risk behaviors among bisexual and homosexual adolescents. *Journal of Adolescent Health*, 23(2), 181-188.

Sechrist, W. (2000). Health educators and child maltreatment: A curious silence. *Journal of School Health*, 70(6), 241-243.

Sexuality Information and Health Council of the United States (SIECUS). 1996. *Guidelines for comprehensive sexuality education, 2nd edition*. New York: Author.

SIECUS. (1999). Public support for sexuality education reaches highest level, survey says. *SHOP Talk*, June 11, Vol. 4, Issue 7. Online at http://www.siecus.org/pubs/shop/volume4/shpv40022.html

SIECUS. (2001). Sexuality education for people with disabilities. *SIECUS Report*, Volume 29, Number 3.

Solomon, J., and Card, J.J. (2004) *Making the List: Understanding, Selecting, and Replicating EffectiveTeen Pregnancy Prevention Programs*. Washington, DC: National Campaign to Prevent Teen Pregnancy.

Thornberry, T. Wei, E., Stouthamer-Loeber, M., & Van Dyke, J. (2000). *Teenage fatherhood and delinquent behavior*. Washington, DC: Office of Juvenile Justice and Delinquency Prevention. (http://ojjdp.ncjrs.org/pubs/delinqsum.html#178899)

U.S. Department of Education Office for Civil Rights. (1992) *Teenage pregnancy and parenthood issues (under Title IX of the Education Amendments of 1972). (Code No.20)*. Washington, DC: Author.

U.S. Department of Education Office for Civil Rights. (1999). *Protecting students from harassment and hate crime: A guide for schools*. Washington, DC: Author.

U.S. Department of Education & U.S. Department of Justice. (1998). *Safe and smart: Making after-school hours work for kids.* Available at: http://www.ed.gov/21stcclc/.

U.S. Department of Education & U.S. Department of Justice. (2000). *Working for children and families: Safe and smart after-school programs.* Washington, DC: Authors.

U.S. Department of Health and Human Services. (1995). *Adolescent time use, risky behavior, and outcomes: An analysis of national data.* Washington, DC: Author.

U.S. Department of Health and Human Services. (2000a). *Healthy people 2010: Understanding and improving health.* Washington, DC: U.S. Department of Health and Human Services, Government Printing Office.

U.S. Department of Health and Human Services. (2000b). Standards for privacy of individually identifiable health information: Final Rule, *Federal Register.* 65(250), December 28. Washington, DC: National Archives and Records Administration.

U.S. Department of Health and Human Services. (2002). Modifications to the standards for privacy of individually identifiable health information—Final Rule. *HHS Fact Sheet.* Online: www.hhs.gov/news/press/2002pres/20020809.html.

Virginia Department of Education. (1991). *Family life education: Effective instruction for students in special education.* Richmond, VA: Author.

Washington State Department of Health. (1999). *Lessons learned: Five years of teen pregnancy prevention community projects.* Olympia, WA: Author.

Whitaker, D.J., Miller, K.S., May, D.C., & Levin, M.L. (1999). Teenage partners' communication about sexual risk and condom use: The importance of parent-teenager discussions. *Family Planning Perspectives*, 31(3), 117-121.

The White House Office of National AIDS Policy. (2000). *Youth and AIDS 2000: A new American agenda.* Washington, DC: Author. Available at http://www.whitehouse.gov/ONAP/youth_report1.pdf

Wiley, D.C. & Terlosky, B. (2000). Evaluating sexuality education curriculums. *Educational Leadership*, 58:2, 79-82.

Wolf, W.C. (1999). *Using Title IX to protect the rights of pregnant and parenting teens.* Bala Cynwyd, PA: Center for Assessment and Policy Development. Available online at http://www.capd.org/home/services/teenparents/ta_adds/weblist13.pdf